AUTOPHAGY

Purify your body, promote muscle growth, slow aging and lose weight easily, through targeted diets

Michaela Hampton

© **Copyright 2019 by Michaela Hampton**
All rights reserved.

This document is geared towards providing exact and reliable information with regards to the topic and issue covered. The publication is sold with the idea that the publisher is not required to render accounting, officially permitted, or otherwise, qualified services. If advice is necessary, legal or professional, a practiced individual in the profession should be ordered.

-From a Declaration of Principles which was accepted and approved equally by a Committee of the American Bar Association and a Committee of Publishers and Associations.

In no way is it legal to reproduce, duplicate, or transmit any part of this document in either electronic means or in printed format. Recording of this publication is strictly prohibited and any storage of this document is not allowed unless with written permission from the publisher. All rights reserved.

The information provided herein is stated to be truthful and consistent, in that any liability, in terms of inattention or otherwise, by any usage or abuse of any policies, processes or directions contained within is the solitary and utter responsibility of the recipient reader. Under no circumstances will any legal responsibility or blame beheld against the publisher for any reparation, damages, or monetary loss due to the information herein, either directly or indirectly.

Respective authors own all copyrights not held by the publisher.

The information herein is offered for informational purposes solely, and is universal as saw. The presentation of the information is without contract or any type of guarantee assurance.

The trademarks that are used are without any consent, and the publication of the trademark is without permission or backing by the trademark owner. All trademarks and brands within this book are for clarifying purposes only and are the owned by the owners themselves, not affiliated with this document.

Contents

- THEORIES OF AGING 5
- DEACIDIFY, PURIFY BE HEALTHY 22
- WHAT IS AUTOPHAGY? 36
- AUTOPHAGY: "SELF-MUTILATION" AS A SURVIVAL STRATEGY 40
- AUTOPHAGY: HOW DOES IT WORK? 44
- ADVANTAGES OF AUTOPHAGY 45
- THIS WILL GET MORE AUTOPHAGIA IN YOUR LIFE 48
- WHAT CONTROLS AUTOPHAGY? 52
- WHAT ARE THE TASKS OF AUTOPHAGY? 53
- THE PLACE OF AUTOPHAGY 57
- AUTOPHAGY ENDOGENOUS RECYCLING 62
- THE DIFFERENT PROCESSES OF AUTOPHAGY 65
- SELF-HEALING THROUGH A FUNCTIONING AUTOPHAGY 71
- AUTOPHAGY ACTIVATION0/TRIGGER 75
- WHAT IS FASTING? 79
- WHAT IS INTERMITTENT FASTING? 81
- THE BENEFITS OF INTERMITTENT FASTING 84
- WHY YOU SHOULD FAST REGULARLY 86
- WEIGHT LOSS 92
- ARE ALL CALORIES THE SAME? 101
- MACRONUTRIENTS 105
- WHAT INTERVAL FAST VARIANTS ARE THERE? 113
- INTERVAL FASTING: INSTRUCTIONS FOR THE 16/8 VARIANT 117
- NUTRITION PLANS FOR INTERMITTENT FASTING 120
- INTERMITTENT FASTING: LEANGAINS METHOD 132
- 16: 8 INTERVAL FASTING: THE 8-HOUR DIET 138
- AUTOPHAGY RECYCLING AND SURVIVAL 141

- AUTOPHAGY HELPS FIGHT ALZHEIMER'S ... 145
- KETOGENIC DIET AND INTERVAL FASTING ... 147
- WHAT AFFECTS AUTOPHAGY? ... 152
- ALL THE BENEFITS OF KETOGENIC NUTRITION AT A GLANCE ... 156
- STRENGTHEN MITOCHONDRIA: CELL TRAINING FOR MORE ENERGY ... 163
- CIRCADIAN RHYTHM ... 172
- RECIPES ... 180
- DESSERT ... 191

THEORIES OF AGING

There are hundreds of theories that try to explain aging.

Several mechanisms have already been scientifically investigated, which describe the aging of the cells of the human organism. These include, for example, gene regulation theory, DNA damage repair theory, mitochondrial aging, and so on.

Specific theories assume that aging is genetically predestined, and other explanations lead to aging back to signs of erosion. By way of example, the theory of the telomeres, which has a genetic background, and the theory of free radicals (oxidative stress), which is to be found in the case of wear and tear, are listed here.

1. The theory of telomeres

This theory assumes that the number of cell divisions and the number of regeneration processes are limited. The chromosomes in the nucleus, which contain the genetic material in the form of DNA strands - packed in proteins - have particularly stable ends. These ends are called telomeres. They represent protective caps for the chromosomes.

With each cell division, the two DNA strands of a chromosome separate and double again. The enzymes that accomplish this doubling, shed a bit at the end of the DNA strands with each cell division.

At the beginning of cell divisions, according to this theory, neither the cell nor the genes are damaged. Because the ends of the DNA strands - the telomeres - contain no genetic information. But after a while, the clipped areas do not just extend to the telomeres, but genes are also affected. The cell loses its functionality. When the telomeres were lost, it could be observed in experiments that the chromosomes joined together, changed their structure, and otherwise behaved abnormally.

Preservation and a flawless transfer of genetic information were no longer guaranteed. Thus, the cell is doomed. In this context, one speaks of programmed cell death.

2. Free radicals (oxidative stress)

The so-called "free radicals" are very reactive molecules. They have a free electron and therefore make straightforward connections. These molecules are formed, for example, in the normal combustion process in the cell.

But external influences, such as UV light or radioactivity, favor the formation of reactive molecules, as well as smoking.

Chemically, these are usually reactive oxygen atoms, oxygen-nitrogen radicals, hydrogen peroxide, and hydroxyl groups. In each cell, over 10,000 of these highly reactive compounds are formed daily. Of course, the cells have repair mechanisms that repair the cell damage caused by the radicals. But at some point, the battery is so attacked that it is no longer functional.

When cell death occurs, depending on the cell type, then the effects are felt. The skin becomes gray and wrinkled and connective tissue cells, the muscles, are less convincing when the they are affected.

Aging, a unique human problem. This definition of aging is quite a mouthful, but it also contains all the necessary keywords that belong to aging. Firstly, aging is characterized by changes that take place in the organism. Secondly, the effects of these changes are becoming increasingly visible over time.

Thirdly, changes, and their effects on functioning make the aging individual more sensitive to the causes of death. The risk of death, therefore, increases with age. Finally, despite the fact that aging comes from the inside, as it were, there is an interaction with the external causes of death, such as infectious diseases or complications after an accident.

Some organisms do not age

An important complication in studying aging is that the process is gradual. Changes are often subtle and cannot always be recognized overnight. At the same time, changes due to aging are often arbitrary. The challenge is to recognize the relevant changes therein.

To determine whether a species (or organism) ages, you can fortunately also measure something simple - the risk of death, or vice versa - the survival in groups of the species in question. This is called a cohort. In an organism that does not age, the chance of dying is independent of age, and therefore, remains the same with aging. That chance is determined by the environment, for example, by predators.

Conversely, the chance of dying increases with age in an organism where aging is part of the biology of the species. So, even though aging affects the functioning of the individual, measuring all kinds of biological and demographic aspects of the aging process is often the most effective in groups of individuals, in cohorts.

To study the aging process, you must distinguish between intrinsic and extrinsic causes of death; in other words, mortality due to aging or environmental factors.

Survival and stiffness in human populations

This cahier is not about lifespan and death in fruit flies, but about human aging. More specifically, it is about the causes and consequences of the spectacular increase in the life expectancy of people and what this has for individual, collective, and societal consequences.

In the past, you often died from environmental causes, now more and more often from aging. It may sound surprising, but the situation for the fruit flies from the graphs above also applied to humans for a long time. Around 1800, mortality was still determined by environmental causes, the "environmental mortality." Around 1980, this role was almost completely taken over by aging mortality. About 200 years ago, the causes of environmental mortality were as diverse as limited food quantity, quality and safety, poor living conditions, insufficient hygiene, poor nutrition, and no knowledge of important pathogens such as bacteria and viruses.

Improved hygiene, medical care, social changes, and scientific insights have largely eliminated these causes of death. This results in a shift in the graph that is comparable to moving the fruit flies from the wild to the laboratory. This shift in mortality from extrinsic to intrinsic factors reduced overall mortality, resulting in an increase in average human life expectancy. In a recent analysis, demographers show how special this increase is and how quickly it has taken place. The decrease in environmental mortality occurred in just four of the estimated 8,000 generations that Homo sapiens has known so far.

The increase in our life expectancy is, therefore, the result of the fact that we humans have changed our own environment in such a way that the potential for aging and longevity can be expressed. This, and the speed with which life expectancy has risen in two hundred years, excludes that genetic changes have contributed to this.

Variation in aging in human populations

Answering the question "Why?" also gives entry to the "How?" and other mechanistic questions about the biology of aging. The boxes between the chapters of this booklet tell how different parts of our body age. The basic idea of accumulation of damage, with catastrophic consequences for the functioning of the individual organism (read: death), for example, can easily be explained by the current evolutionary theories of aging.

It is important to map, study, and, above all, understand the mechanisms of human aging. With that, you can also understand something about the variation in health, life span, and aging in human populations. Because the average life expectancy may increase, it does not alter the fact that there is still great variation in the lifespan of individuals. Which factors contribute to this variation?

The course of life expectancy in human populations already showed the strong influence of the environment. The healthier the environment, the longer we lived. Still, the variation in income, living conditions, and lifestyle are strongly related to life expectancy.

But recent estimates in twin populations also show that about twenty-percent (20%) of the current variation in life expectancy is due to genetic variation. There are families in which many people are getting very old. The brother of a hundred-year-old sometimes has an eight times greater chance of turning one hundred than his peers. A lot of such long-lived families have also been found in the in Europe. That is why the following wisdom often goes around in the literature on aging: *"If you want to live long, choose your parents well!"*

There is a third factor that is important for explaining variation in lifespan in human populations – the interaction between the environment and genetic variation. After all, the above analysis of the increase in human life expectancy shows that this increase is not the result of genetic changes.

In other words, our genome, our genetic composition, and how it makes our body function, was once selected in a very different environment from where we now live. The fundamental idea of evolutionary adaptation through natural selection is that there is an optimal connection between the genome and the environment.

But the rapid change of our environment, caused by our own actions in only the last four of 8,000 generations of modern humans, cannot be followed by an appropriate response from our genes. The process of natural selection is simply too slow for that; it requires more than four generations.

The big difference between our evolutionary environment and our contemporary environment is the pressure of infectious diseases and the amount of food composition. This "evolutionary mismatch" could very well underlie the increased frequency of autoimmune diseases, heart disease, obesity, and type 2 diabetes. In particular, the realization that the interaction between genes and the environment can be important for life expectancy and health gives people the opportunity to actively influence health through influencing their personal environment; for example, through nutrition.

Mutation Accumulation

The first modern theory of mammalian aging was formulated by Peter Medawar in 1952. It formed from discussions in the previous decade with JBS Haldane and the selection shadow concept. Their idea was that aging was a matter of neglect. Nature is a very competitive place, and almost all animals in nature die before they reach old age. Therefore, there is not much reason why the body must stay fit for the long term - not much selection pressure for traits that would maintain viability beyond the time when most animals would be killed; killed by predators, disease, or accident.

Medawar theory is referred to as *Mutation accumulation.* The mechanism of action includes random, harmful *germline* mutations of a species that happen to show their effect in life. Unlike the most harmful mutations, these would not be efficiently eradicated by natural selection. On a large scale, aging would simply be the addition of harmful genes that are only present in older individuals. Hence, they would "accumulate," and perhaps, because of all that decay and damage that we associate with aging.

Modern genetics science has described a potential problem with the mutation accumulation concept that it is now known that genes are typically expressed in specific tissues at specific times. The expression is controlled by a number of genetic "programs" that activate different genes at different times in the normal growth, development, and day-to-day life of the organism. Defects in the genes lead to problems (genetic diseases), when not properly expressed when needed. A problem later in life suggests that the genetic program called for expression of a gene that occurs only at a later age and mutation defect prevents proper expression. This implies the existence of a program called different gene expressions at that point in life. Why, given Medawar's understanding, would there exist genes only needed in later life or a program only called in later life for different expressions? The *maintenance mechanism* theory (discussed below) prevents this problem.

The Medawar concept has suggested that the evolutionary process was influenced by the age at which an organism was able to reproduce. Traits that negatively affected an organism prior to that age would severely limit the organism's ability to propagate its characteristics, and thus, would be "selected on the basis of" natural selection. Properties that propagate the same adverse effects that only turned out well after that age would have caused relatively little effect on the ability of the organism, and therefore, could be allowed through natural selection. This concept fits well with the observed multitude of mammalian lifespan (and varying ages in sexual maturity) and is important to all subsequent theories of aging discussed below.

The role of extrinsic death rates

Young cohorts, in numbers not yet exhausted by extrinsic death rates, contribute much more to the next generation than the few remaining older cohorts; so the power of selection against late-acting harmful mutations, which only affect these few older people, is very weak. The mutations cannot be selected by then and can spread over the evolutionary time in the population.

The most important testable prediction made by this model is that species that have high extrinsic death rates in nature age much faster and have a shorter intrinsic lifespan. This is confirmed among the mammals, the best studied in terms of life history. There is a correlation between mammals between body size and lifespan so that larger species live longer than smaller species under controlled/optimal conditions, but there are exceptions. For example, many bats and rodents are of similar size, but bats live much longer.

For example, the small brown bat, half the size of a mouse, can live 30 years in the wild. A mouse will only live 2-3 years, even under optimum conditions. The explanation is that bats have fewer predators, and therefore low extrinsic mortality. More people survive until later age, so the power of selection against late-acting harmful mutations is stronger. Fewer working harmful mutations mean lower mortality, and therefore, a longer lifespan. Birds are also warm-blooded and are similar in size to many small mammals, yet often live 5-10 times as long. They have less predation pressure than ground-living mammals. Seabirds, which in general have the least predators of all birds, live the longest.

When examining the body size versus longevity relationship, It is also noted that predatory mammals tend to live longer than prey mammals in a controlled environment such as a zoo or nature reserve. The explanation for the longevity of primates (such as humans, monkeys, and great apes) relative to body size is that their intelligence, and often their sociality, help them prevent prey. Due to the high position in the food chain, intelligence and cooperativeness all reduce extrinsic mortality rates in species.

Mechanism

If organisms deliberately limit their lifespan through aging or semi-parous behavior, the associated evolved mechanisms can be very complex, just as the mechanisms that provide for laying, vision, digestion, or other biological function are usually very complex. Such a mechanism would typically include hormones, signaling, detection of external conditions, and other complex functions, evolved mechanisms. Such complex mechanisms can explain all observations of aging and semi-porous behavior, as described below.

It is typical for a particular biological function to be controlled by the same mechanism that is capable of perceiving the circumstances and performing the required function. The mechanism signals all systems and tissues that must respond to this function through organism-wide signals (hormones). If aging is indeed a biological function, we would expect all or most manifestations of aging to be controlled in the same way by a common mechanism. Various observations (see below) indeed suggest the existence of a common control mechanism.

It is also typical of biological functions to be modulated by or synchronized with external events or conditions. The circadian rhythm and synchronization of the mating behavior of planetary signals are examples. When aging as a biological function, the calorific restriction effect can also be an example of the aging function modulated in order to optimize organism lifespan in response to external conditions. Temporary extension of lifespan under famine would help the survival group because extended lifespan, combined with less frequent reproduction, would be required to maintain resources in a particular population.

Theories about the effect that aging results as standard (mutation accumulation), or is a negative side effect of another function, are logically much more limited and suffer compared to empirical evidence for complex mechanisms. The choice of the parent theory, therefore, logically essentially determined by the point of view regarding evolutionary processes, and some theorists reject programmed aging based entirely on evolutionary process considerations.

Maintenance Theories

It is generally accepted that deteriorating processes (wear and tear, other molecular damage) exist and that living organisms have mechanisms to prevent deterioration – heal wounds, dead cells are replaced, or claws grow back.

A non-programmed theory of mammalian aging that fits into modern evolutionary theory and the Medawar concept is that different mammalian species have different options for maintenance and repair. Longer living species have many mechanisms for compensating for damage due to causes such as oxidation, telomere shortening and other deteriorating processes that are each more effective than those of the shorter life species. Shorter living species, with earlier centuries of sexual maturity, had less need for a long life and therefore did not evolve or retain the more effective recovery mechanisms. Damage therefore accumulates faster, causing earlier revelations and a shorter lifespan.

A corresponding programmed maintenance theory based on evolvability suggests that the recovery mechanisms are in turn controlled by a common operating mechanism to detect suitable states, such as calorific limitation, and also be able to have the specific lifespan required for the particular species. In this view, the differences between the short and long life are species in the control mechanisms, as opposed to each individual maintenance mechanism.

DNA damage theory of aging

The DNA damage theory of aging is an important explanation for aging at the molecular level. This theory postulates that DNA damage is ubiquitous in the biological world and is the leading cause of aging. In accordance with this theory, genetic elements that regulate the repair of DNA damage in somatic cells were suggested to have pleiotropic effects that are beneficial during early development but allow harmful effects later in life. As an example, studies of brain and muscle mammals have shown that DNA repair ability is relatively high during early development when cells divide mitotically but decreases substantially as cells invade post-mitotic states. The reduction in DNA repair capacity presumably reflects an evolutionary adaptation to divert the means of cell duplication and repairs to more essential neuronal and muscle functions. Reduction in expression of DNA repair capacity has increased accumulation of DNA damage. This then impairs gene transcription and causes the progressive loss of cellular and tissue functions to define aging.

Evidence

Complex programmed death mechanisms exist in semelparous species (e.g. octopus), including hormone signaling, involvement of the nervous system, etc. If a limited life span is generally useful as predicted by the programmed aging theories, it would be unusual for an octopus to possess a more complex mechanism for accomplishing that function than a mammal.

"Aging genes" without other identifiable function. But to date no evidence that such genes exist has been found.

Calorie reduction effect: reducing the available resources increases the lifespan. This behavior has a plausible group benefit in improving the survival of a famine group and also suggests common control.

Progeria and Werner syndrome both single-gene genetic diseases that cause acceleration of many or most symptoms of aging. The fact that a single gene defect can have similar effects on many manifestations of aging suggests a common mechanism. However, both genes influenced DNA stability and thus can be explained by stochastic theories of aging that attribute aging accumulation of DNA damage.

Although mammalian lifetimes vary over an approximately 100: 1 range, manifestations of aging (cancer, arthritis, weakness, sensory, etc.) are similar in different types. This suggests that the deterioration of the mechanisms and associated maintenance mechanisms work over a short period (less than the life span of a short-lived mammal). All mammals must therefore have all the maintenance mechanisms. This suggests the difference between mammals in a control mechanism or repair efficiency.

Lifespan differs considerably from different-looking species (for example, different species of salmon 3: 1, different fish 600: 1) suggests that relatively few genes have a lifetime and that relatively small changes to genotype can cause large differences in lifetime. This would be consistent with a common lifespan control mechanism, but bear in mind that this in itself does not provide evidence of programmed aging, but is also consistent with traditional theories.

DEACIDIFY, PURIFY BE HEALTHY

♦♦♦

Deacidification is one of the most critical steps on the way to health. How to properly deacidify the body, one believes long to know. And yet, after some acidification treatments, the results are not infrequent. The reason: Many deacidification treatments deacidify the gastrointestinal tract. But they do not deacidify the tissue, and they certainly do not deacidify the cell itself.

Deacidify and purify

Deacidification is a lifestyle today. Because deacidification is essential - at least when modern living and eating are modern. Ready meals, sausages, cheeses, snacks, sweets, soft drinks, caffeine, nicotine, and alcohol are now part of everyday life, but all of them acidify the organism. Similarly, environmental toxins, heavy metals, and poisons from textiles or building materials acidify. Stress, bullying, and strife eventually overflow the acid barrel called man. As a result, much and often, but not correctly, is deacidified.

Deacidification - an unfulfilled dream?

Usually, a healthy body can regularly deacidify and detoxify itself - without the human being having to intervene here. Today, however, the detoxification and purification capacities of the organism are often overburdened. So, the body can usually no longer neutralize on its own.

For autonomous deacidification, he lacks the basic requirements of a healthy lifestyle such as exercise, sunlight, micronutrients, relaxation, water, harmony, and - most importantly - an elemental diet. Deacidification, therefore, remains an unfulfilled dream for many people, and the acids and slags remain in the intercellular tissue. However, the intercellular fabric has the task of supplying and disposing of the cells.

One can imagine the intercellular tissue as a supermarket for the cells with the attached waste disposal plant. Cells receive everything they need from intercellular tissue: glucose, oxygen, vitamins, amino acids, fatty acids, minerals, etc.

At the same time, they permanently release their waste, including acids, to the intercellular tissue. The intercellular fabric is thus dependent on an agile transport mechanism. Nutrients and micronutrients must be produced, and waste must be transported away.

If not deacidified, the cell suffocates

If there is acidification, the intercellular tissue is used as a reservoir for acids and slags. This causes the river to falter. Waste can no longer be wholly removed and remains lying, which aggravates the acidification and slagging.

At some point there is hardly any room left for other waste, including acids. The cells do not know what to do with their garbage and have to store it in their interior. As a result, the cell itself now too acidifies.

In a sluggish intercellular tissue, of course, at the same time, the nutrient supply is at risk. For how should nutrients and micronutrients find their way to the cells when the intercellular tissue is full of slags and acids? Not only does the cell suffocate almost from its waste, but it also hardly receives the much-needed nutrients.

The cell lives like a slum. She is hungry and surrounded by garbage. Understandable, when she gets angry.

Acidification makes you sick and ugly

But slurred and over-acidified intercellular tissue, together with malnourished and acidic cells, is the prerequisite for everything we really do not want:

- Overweight
- Cellulite
- Varicose veins
- Spider veins
- Impure or gray skin
- Hair loss
- Brittle fingernails
- Joint pain
- Dental and gum problems
- Bad eyes
- Lack of concentration and much more
- Deacidification makes you healthy and attractive

What we would like to have would be here:
- Ideal weight
- Smooth and flawless skin
- Healthy blood vessels
- Full and healthy hair
- Strong fingernails
- Movable joints
- Healthy teeth until old age

- Sharp view
- Ability to concentrate and many more positive things
- Magic word deacidifying the body

Deacidification is the magic word. This is nothing new anymore. Therefore, half of the world is currently deacidified - mostly in the following way:

A base powder is used to provide the organism with sufficient minerals that it needs to neutralize the acids that accumulate and to provide the resulting slags for disposal.

Base baths are used to excrete slag and acids through the skin. Also, brush massages are performed to stimulate deacidification via the lymph.

It turns the diet on a basic diet, avoid acidifying foods, and preferably alkaline foods. It is dedicated to moderate exercise. You try to avoid stress.

If deacidification fails:

Of course, these measures are already outstanding. Nevertheless, success is too often limited or even completely absent. Why? At points 2 to 5, there is nothing to complain about. They not only support effective deacidification but are also a prerequisite for preventing further unwanted acids from entering the body. But there are two serious problems that prevent deacidification.

Deacidification requires basic nutrition

Problem 1: The diet is usually only slightly changed. On the one hand, because habits are difficult to change. On the other hand, because the right information and the right motivation are missing. Special detoxification treatment is ideal for getting into the right base excess diet. With such a detoxification cure over four weeks, you can easily learn to change your eating habits and receive a variety of suitable recipes.

You can feast basically

Find out more about the varied basic breakfast and get to know the healthy deacidified alkaline cakes. Experiment with basic spreads, basic potato dishes, and basic snacks. Immerse yourself in the basic world of crisp, healthy sprouts. And if you want to get to know the ultimate in basic lifestyles, then you should learn about green smoothies.

Deacidification requires high-quality base preparations

Problem 2: However, the measures mentioned above alone are often not enough to successfully deacidify. In many cases, they no longer manage to deacidify the organism and especially the cell interior. For this reason, a base preparation (point 1) is always prescribed for deacidification cures.

Acidification of the cells

Many base preparations often deacidify only the gastrointestinal tract, but not the tissue and not the cell itself. So, the slag and many acids remain largely in the body. The hyperacidity does not only take place in the gastrointestinal tract, where it can be relatively easily neutralized with the mentioned minerals. Hyperacidity also takes place directly in the cell - with devastating effects.

You have to know:

- ✓ A basic (= healthy) cell is negatively charged.

- ✓ An acidified (= sick) cell is positively charged.

- ✓ As with iron magnets with north and south poles, it behaves with electromagnetic charges: same poles/charges repel each other, different poles/charges attract.

- ✓ The nutrition of the cell takes place by electromagnetic means.

- ✓ Nutrients that the cell needs are positively charged.

- ✓ If the cell is basic = healthy = negatively charged, it can attract nutrients and thus feed and produce energy.

- ✓ If the cell is acid = sick = positively charged, it repels nutrients, so it can no longer feed, cannot produce energy, the body decays.

An acidic cell can be given as much base powder or nutrients as you want - it simply cannot absorb the minerals or nutrients. Deacidification does not take place; a therapeutic success remains.

Deacidify the cell

However, there is a way out. The cell can now be quickly and effectively freed from its acid reaction rigidity and converted into a basic living state - with the alkaline active water concentrate active bases.

In addition, one must know again:

The positive charge of an acidified cell is due to a high concentration of $H+$ ions.

Water (H_2O) is a molecule and consists of 2 hydrogen atoms (2 times H) and 1 oxygen atom (1 time O), hence the name H_2O.

Now you can also convert water into an ionic form. For this, one needs strong electric current, salt, and other special technological conditions. Then, you get positively charged $H+$ ions (per molecule of water) and negatively charged $OH-$ ions (also per molecule of water). This is still water, but it now has a lot of electrical potentials and ... it's very basic.

Deacidification with active bases

The name of this water is "active bases." If you drink this water, then these H + and OH - ions float around in the intercellular tissue, i.e., in the fluid that surrounds the cells. The positively charged H + ions are repelled by the positively charged, but acidified cell, but the negatively charged OH ions are attracted and can enter the cell.

Deacidify every single cell

Now the fascinating thing happens. Part of the penetrating negative OH ions combines with the positive H + ions (which are inside the cell) to form water. The other part brings the cell into a negatively charged, i.e., basic state. The newly created water now flooded the accumulated garbage out of the cell, while the cell at the same time by the negative charge again nutrients attract and can also absorb, because only now - since the garbage was taken out - even more, space for nutrients.

The cell no longer has to live in filth and hunger. She is well looked after again and clean around her. The gloomy slum became a pretty residential area.

Deacidified with active bases

Active bases is a concentrate with a pH between 10.5 and 11. Therefore it is taken in small amounts and diluted with water.

Directions for use: Twice a day, add 25 milliliters in about 150 milliliters of water (which is a small glass), and drink about 1 hour before a meal.

Deacidification with active bases should be carried out purely prophylactically twice a year. In case of complaints more often, in order to give the cells sufficient opportunity actually to leave the acidic state of the reaction rigidity.

Learn now how to properly and successfully deacidify. We will also introduce you to four acidification treatments - the right one for every person, every condition, and every everyday life. Two of them are based on active bases and are especially recommended for those people who have been acidified for a long time and finally want to find a way out:

The deacidification program

Carry out a 1 to 3-month deacidification program, e.g., B. with basic active water concentrate (active bases). These programs allow both extra- and intracellular deacidification. As part of a high-quality deacidification treatment - depending on the selected cure - you will be accompanied by other components that accelerate and intensify the deacidification. Basic baths, bitter substances, liquid bentonite, basic tea, etc.

If you find that the daily time spent on such a complete program seems too high, but you still want to deacidify, then you can opt for the simplest, yet successful method of deacidification with active bases. Active bases is a basic active water concentrate that can deacidify the body down to the cell level. In the case of acid-base deacidification, you only have to think about taking active bases twice a day. That's all.

Eat base excess - even AFTER your 1 to 3-month detoxification treatment. The cure was only the entry! Those slags that have been in your body for many years can often only be eliminated after several months of basic life. In addition, you must also consistently withdraw the always new incoming acids or those that result from mental or physical stress.

If you still want to eat acidifying unhealthy food now and then, you must regularly provide your organism with high-quality alkaline minerals (e.g., a vegetable base powder, a citrate mix, or the Sango Marine Coral) to remove as many acids as possible can. Any change towards a healthy diet increases the chances of daily complete slag disposal.

- ✓ Include the following points (or at least some of them) in your future daily routine:

- ✓ Start the day with a basic morning tea.

- ✓ Use basic body care products as basic as possible (see basic body care, e.g., a basic shower gel, a basic shampoo, etc.)

- ✓ If you are in a hurry in the morning, have breakfast with a quick-prepared based cereal.

- ✓ To supplement your diet with high-quality basic substances, you can sprinkle a vegetable base powder over each meal.

- ✓ Organic basic minerals such. For example, the Sango Marine Coral is regularly ingested so that the body can finally return all the minerals it has borrowed from its mineral deposits during the depletion.

- ✓ Relax at least two to three times a week in a base bath. If you do not have time for a full bath, you should treat yourself to basic foot baths.

- ✓ Pay attention to deep, conscious breathing.

- ✓ Plan moderate sports and sauna visits in your weekly routine.

- ✓ In the evening you enjoy basic evening tea.

- ✓ In natural medicine, it is also assumed that you can also deacidify well on the soles and therefore recommends base stockings that are worn at night and continue to deacidify in your sleep.

- ✓ Check your deacidification success with the Sander acid-base test.

The acid-base test shows the degree of hyperacidity

Before a base therapy (deacidification), you can determine the degree of hyperacidity with the help of an acid-base test. In this way, it is much easier to assess whether and in what form deacidification is required.

WHAT IS AUTOPHAGY?

♦ ♦ ♦

The body is not a rigid structure, but a highly complex and dynamic masterpiece. Construction and dismantling always take place in parallel, also parallel in the same line. The degradation can be done thoroughly; the utilization of carbohydrates and fats to CO_2, water, and energy in the form of ATP is known. The incomplete degradation of complex molecules into the individual components is often overlooked:

During autophagy, the cell degrades parts of the cell interior is tiny drops of fat (vesicles), and from them, extracts new building blocks (amino acids, sugars, nucleotides,).

These fat droplets are referred to herein as autophagosomes.

The term *autophagy* is composed of *auto* (Greek for self) and phagocytosis ("cell eating"). Colloquially, the cell partly eats/digests itself. However, this has little to do with suicide, more with recycling: Autophagy contributes to the breakdown of old and damaged cell components and is essential for keeping the cell young and vital 1,9.

Autophagy is possible in every single cell in the body, but it also takes place outside the battery in the immune system : In fasted states in which autophagy is activated, macrophages circulate throughout the body, increasingly looking for infected cells, dead cells and pathogens, If you are sick in bed with flu, your body suppresses feelings of hunger to activate autophagy, which helps fight the infection.

A special form is a pinocytosis: This instrument, also known as "cell-drinking," is used by the cell to absorb, recycle, and self-use new cell material from lymph in large quantities.

Autophagy translates with self-digestion. It refers to a process in living cells in which cell components are broken down and utilized. At least 35 genes control the complex regulated process. For many decades, the autophagy has been explored by, among others, the Japanese molecular biologist Yoshinori Ohsumi. In October 2016, he received the Nobel Prize for Medicine for his work.

The autophagy proceeds as follows: First, the cell lays a unique sheath around the components that are to be broken down. The sheath closes to the autophagosome. This then fuses with lysosomes; these are small bubbles full of enzymes. The enzymes have the ability to break down and break down the components included in the shell. For example, it creates amino acids and lipids that can be newly installed or used for energy. The body identifies other degradation products as waste; they have transported away and excreted.

Autophagy is mainly triggered when the supply of nutrients stops. A situation that arises, for example, during fasting or intense sports. In this situation of deficiency, the cell relies on its resources. It breaks down what is not needed and thus gains new nutrients and energy. For self-digestion, the body dissects dead cell components, faulty proteins, and even whole-cell organelles, such as older mitochondria. Even pathological or potentially pathogenic structures, as well as invading bacteria and viruses, are disposed of. Therefore, autophagy is often described as a process of self-purification and self-preservation. It has evolved in the course of evolution to eliminate defective structures while conserving energy and nutrients.

In contrast to the natural renewal of body cells and organs, autophagy is much faster and more flexible. It can provide cell renewal virtually daily, while a real rejuvenation of cells can take days to years.

Autophagy also plays a role in the fight against infections and stress, as well as in embryonic development, to quickly have the required building blocks ready. Since a temporary energy deficit favors autophagy, it can be activated by fasting. This is another explanation for the positive health effects caused by regular fasting.

AUTOPHAGY:
"SELF-MUTILATION" AS A SURVIVAL STRATEGY

♦ ♦ ♦

In nature, nothing is lost: both for living things and for the entire biosphere, processes are characteristic in which a large part of the starting materials is recovered. One such regulation of the human cell is autophagy - a recycling program that allows it to break down damaged or misfolded proteins down to whole organelles and then reuse them.

The phenomenon of autophagy was first described in the 1960s. For a long time, only a small group of researchers devoted themselves to this area. This has changed in recent years. Now the importance of this important cell process is reflected in the Nobel Prize Committee's recognition: The Japanese Yoshinori Ohsumi is honored for his discoveries of autophagy mechanisms. His work "has dramatically changed the understanding of this vital process," says the Nobel Prize committee's rationale.

With the crucial experiments, Ohsumi started in the early 1990s on yeast cells (Saccharomyces cerevisiae). At that time, it was already known that certain organelles, the lysosomes, degrade cellular components. The Belgian Christian de Duve had already received the Nobel Prize in 1974. It was he who coined the term autophagy.

But it was not until Ohsumi's work that it became clear which processes were going to be exactly the same and how important they are for human health. With a series of sophisticated experiments, he showed that 15 genes are involved in autophagy. Using his research, he described the network of signals and proteins that control the process in its various stages.

Cellular recycling: a highly complex process

Recycling is a matter of course for cells - the molecular waste is precisely packed by a membrane and sent to the lysosomes for recycling. In this highly complex process (graphic)Cell components that are no longer performing their task properly are channeled into the interior of autophagosomes. These are vesicles with a double membrane, which include proteins, lipids, membrane components, and whole organelles (mitochondria) from the cytoplasm into their interior. The autophagosomes then merge with lysosomes to autophagolysosomes, where the particles are degraded by acid hydrolases, and their basic building blocks are made available for recycling. Ultimately, this mechanism helps to keep the degradation of old and the production of new cell components in balance (cellular homeostasis).

Autophagy is continuously active at a basal level but is specifically activated in stressful situations. In extreme situations, such as severe cell damage, either apoptosis or so-called autophagosomal cell death - a non-apoptotic, programmed cell death - can be initiated. Autophagy is thus a mechanism for survival of the individual cell, but also a suicide program for damaged cells to ensure the survival of a multicellular organism. It is therefore easy to understand that a dysregulated or diminished autophagic activity, as we presumably find it in old age, inevitably leads to a cellular disaster that manifests itself in a whole range of diseases.

These include:

- Cancer (lack of tumor suppression, dysregulated cell death, lack of elimination of damaged organelles),

- Accumulation of neurodegenerative plaques in dementia (impaired intracellular protein degradation),

- Muscular diseases (neuromuscular syndromes, myopathies),
- Infectious diseases (disturbed autophagosomal elimination of intracellular pathogens),
- functional hepatic insufficiency.

Autophagy: what do you have?

Autophagy plays a role, among other things, in the normal functioning of your immune system and in defense of (infectious) diseases. We will tell you more about the benefits of autophagy later in this post.

AUTOPHAGY: HOW DOES IT WORK?

As mentioned earlier, you can stimulate autophagy by doing a detox. More about that later. First autophagy. How does that work?

Your cells make membranes. These membranes look for dead or damaged cells in your body. Their goal is to clean up and reuse these dead or damaged cells, where possible.

Membranes remove the good, yet to be used, parts from a cell and use these parts to make new cell parts.

That is how you clean up old cells in your body with autophagy. Autophagy makes our bodies better-oiled machines.

Autophagy is our body's way of stopping dangerous cell division and resolving issues such as obesity and problems with your metabolism.

ADVANTAGES OF AUTOPHAGY

There are many scientifically-proven benefits of autophagy.

1. CLEAN UP PROTEINS

Research shows that autophagy cleans up the proteins that may cause brain damage. In certain brain disorders, proteins clump together in the body. Autophagy ensures that these clumps can no longer pose a threat.

The clumps are **surrounded by a kind of jacket** (autophagosome). This jacket comes later with another jacket (lysosome) that is full of a digestive enzyme. The clumped proteins are thus rendered harmless.

2. LESS THICK AND BETTER BRAIN

There are indications that rats that are unable to autophagy are fatter and sleepier than their counterparts that are capable of autophagy. Also, they have higher cholesterol and a poorer brain.

- Supplying the cells with molecular building blocks and energy

- Recycling damaged proteins, organelles and aggregates

- Regulatory functions of the mitochondria of cells, which contribute to energy but can be damaged by oxidative stress

- Purification of damaged endoplasmic reticulum and peroxisomes

- Protecting the nervous system and promoting brain and nerve cell growth. Autophagy appears to improve cognitive function, brain structure and neuroplasticity.

- Support the growth of heart cells and protect against heart disease

- Strengthening the immune system by eliminating intracellular pathogens

- Protection against toxic proteins that contribute to a range of amyloid diseases

- Protecting the stability of the DNA

- Prevention of damage to healthy tissues and organs (so-called necrosis)

- Potential fight against cancer, neurodegenerative diseases and other diseases

THIS WILL GET MORE AUTOPHAGIA IN YOUR LIFE

It is good to know that autophagy is your body's response to stress. So, to create some extra autophagy, you have to struggle through some stress.

1. SPORTS

Of course, you have known this for a long time; exercise causes stress. It is not for nothing that you puff and pant and moan and support during boat camps, weightlifting, running, Zumba and cycling.

Regular exercise is **the best way** that people unwittingly help renew their bodies. A study among mice showed that the speed at which the creatures created autophagy increased after they had run on a treadmill for 30 minutes. The speed continued to increase until they were running for 80 minutes.

2. DETOXES

You are fasting with a detox; you do not eat periods. This can be stressful for your body. Your body may not like that at the time of the detox, but in the end, it benefits from this stress because you create autophagy.

Research shows that there are **many benefits of doing a detox,** also called periodic fasting. By regularly doing a detox, you help your body with autophagy.

Other research shows that fasting during a detox improves cognitive functions. Also, fasting would improve neuroplasticity (this helps your brain learn new things).

3. Fewer CARBON HYDRATES

By eating fewer carbohydrates, you relieve your body of its primary source of energy. Normally your body uses carbohydrates. By eating few carbohydrates (50 grams or less), you end up in ketose. Then your body uses fat as fuel instead of carbohydrates.

There are indications that ketosis can help people in **reducing the risk of diabetes.** Also, it is an ideal way to burn fat without losing muscle. For this reason, the ketosis diet is also very popular among bodybuilders.

What boosts autophagy in our cells?

1. Fasting (from about 14 to 17 hours, optimal are regular fasting treatment

2. Calorie restriction (chronic caloric deficit in a balanced diet)

3. Sport (both strength and endurance sports)

4. Some foods and substances: Grazer researchers have been able to identify foods and substances that turn on the cellular garbage disposal, even though the organism eats.

Coffee

Coffee, for example, is an autophagy trigger, the scientists confirm. The tasty pick-me-up is a very popular drink in Germany with a per capita consumption of around 5.5 kg a year. Studies show that coffee has extremely positive effects on various metabolic diseases, such as diabetes or lipid metabolism disorders.

Within one to four hours after the consumption of coffee, there is a strong stimulation of autophagy in all organs examined. This also applies to decaffeinated coffee, that is, it is not due to caffeine, but it is believed that phytochemicals, so-called polyphenols in coffee, have this effect. But beware: animal protein inhibits autophagy again, so do not put cow's milk in the coffee! Only black or with an herbal alternative such. B. Almond milk, coffee promotes self-cleaning of the cells.

WHAT CONTROLS AUTOPHAGY?

Cells do not just eat themselves. This process takes place only under very specific conditions and depends on complex molecular conditions. It involves enzymes such as mTOR and AMPK, which closely monitor how many nutrients and how much energy the cell has available. If there is not enough, they initiate the process of autophagy to break down old cell components that are not currently needed. The resulting components can then be used by the body to build up new and much-needed cell components.

By burning such contaminated sites into usable energy, the body can also guarantee the cell's survival in low-energy phases.

WHAT ARE THE TASKS OF AUTOPHAGY?

1. Autophagy as a survival mechanism

Digesting superfluous waste and using it as a building material or energy → Autophagy serves as a survival mechanism in barren times. Age researcher and Prof. Frank Madeo describes this process in a **lecture on YouTube as** follows: "When cells are exposed to food shortages, they digest everything that is not needed, Cells are able to convert this "cell debris" into energy, which they then re-supply to the body. "

2. Autophagy as part of the immune system and defense mechanism

When foreign proteins or unwanted viruses and bacteria invade the cells, they are simply eaten up by autophagy and rendered harmless.

3. Autophagy as a cleaning-repair mechanism

In the many metabolic processes in our body, it always comes back to damage to cell components and the formation of defective proteins. To prevent them from causing any problems, autophagy simply breaks them down and eliminates them, which in the final stage can also lead to cell death, the so-called apoptosis.

When this purification process is disrupted, more and more substances are deposited in our cells, which is considered to be one of the main causes of cell ageing. One could also say that together with apoptosis, autophagy is the cellular quality control and therefore, essential for maintaining our functionality cells.

In animal experiments, it was shown that calorie reduction increases life expectancy. The reason could be the resulting increased autophagy, through which the cell components are broken down and rebuilt more often so that less "ballast" deposits.

When will autophagy be triggered?

Autophagy occurs to a lesser extent in all cells in the background but is exacerbated by food shortages (especially amino acid deficiency) and any other type of stress (metabolic, genotoxic, infectious and hypoxic).

So, that means fasting and longer periods without food can start the process of autophagy. Researchers have found that we do not have to go hungry for days, but it's enough to fast for 14-18 hours a day, so-called **intermittent fasting.**

During this time, you should refrain from the intake of calories. Drinking water, tea or unsweetened coffee, however, is allowed. Coffee should even accelerate the onset of autophagy.

How to accelerate/amplify autophagy?

Autophagy can be accelerated by drinking coffee during the fasting phase. Apparently, it is not the caffeine that determines the supporting effect, but certain plant substances, so that caffeine-free coffee also works in this regard.

Also advancing autophagy is training during the fasting phase. There is no better way than fasting training to stimulate the purification process of the cells. The movement ultimately increases the energy requirement, and if this is not supplied from outside, cell waste can be particularly effectively recycled and burned to energy.

In addition, spermidine-containing foods such as wheat germ, fresh green pepper, mushrooms, soybean (especially fermented), citrus fruits (especially grapefruit) to promote autophagy.

On the other hand, overeating and high insulin levels inhibit the process of autophagy

- **Supports autophagy:** long breaks between meals (keyword: intermittent fasting)
- Calorie restriction
- Fast
- fasting training
- Coffee
- Spermidine-containing foods
- **Inhibits autophagy too** frequent food
- High insulin levels (keyword: fast-digesting carbohydrates)
- Animal protein
- Sugar, carbohydrates
- Too little movement

Is too much autophagy harmful?

After what has been said so far, it seems sensible to advance the process of autophagy. But autophagy can also be dangerous. In certain tumours, autophagy seems to accelerate the growth of cancer cells. Nevertheless, there is no reason for concern for the average consumer. Autophagy induced by fasting, calorie restriction, coffee, and other measures seems to have a positive effect on longevity and health.

THE PLACE OF AUTOPHAGY

♦ ♦ ♦

The place of autophagy: this is how our cells are built. To understand the process of autophagy as far as possible, it is essential to get an overview of the structure of the cells.

Human cells are considered the smallest functional units of our organism. One can differentiate between cells with one cell nucleus (eucaryotes) and cells without a nucleus (prokaryotes). The typical human cell has a cell nucleus and consists of cytoplasm and the cell membrane as an outer shell. Among other things, the cell maintains its stability via this membrane. It also represents the gatekeeper for various substances. Some hold them back; others let them through into the cell interior. In this context, one speaks of the permeability of the cell.

The nucleus also contains the cell organelles. The nucleus, which is also called a nucleus, contains the genetic information in the form of DNA. A membrane, the nuclear membrane surrounds the cell nucleus itself. The cell organelle mitochondrion is of particular importance because it is considered the powerhouse of the cell. The cell membrane sets the starting point for autophagy, as it begins with certain signals through this recycling process. Another double membrane is created, which later starts with the inclusion of cell waste.

The autophagy in detail

It was the research of the Nobel laureate mentioned above that helped define the processes underlying autophagy. Among other things, the Japanese researcher was able to show that no fewer than 15 genes are involved in the process of autophagy. This also underscores the importance of self-cleaning of cells. The process control of these complex repair measures in the cell takes place, in turn, using specific proteins and signaling substances, which control every single step of the down-conversion process.

The cell begins to move no longer appropriately functioning cell components into the interior of the so-called autophagosomes. The latter is the dual-membrane vesicles already indicated above, which are capable of entrapping proteins, fats, other membrane constituents, or even mitochondria as a whole from within the cytoplasm in their interior.

Like waste in a garbage truck, faulty cell components are shunted into the autophagosome.

Autophagy is part of extensive cellular homeostasis because it helps balance essential cell components. In the process of fusion, autophagosomes, together with lysosomes, develop autophagolysosomes. In this process, the non-functional particles are broken down and converted into building blocks that can be recycled.

The possibilities of autophagy extend to cell death, which is referred to as autophagosomal cell death in comparison to apoptosis or programmed cell death. This cell death is caused by intense stress situations and intense cell damage.

That means autophagy for your health!

Many physicians believe that decreased activity in autophagy increases the risk of certain diseases. These include diabetes, cancer, neurodegenerative diseases, muscle diseases, infectious diseases, and hepatic insufficiency.

The decline in autophagic activity is increasingly associated with aging processes. You can imagine that the cells "waste." So, if you want to avoid severe illnesses in old age, you must necessarily ensure that the "garbage collection" in the cells continues to work well and activate autophagy regularly.

This raises the question of how this can be done effectively. With these tricks, the recycling program of the cells is stimulated.

Some scientists have long been concerned with the question of how to relieve flagellated autophagy. The current state of research highlights the following measures:

Interval fasting.

In particular, targeted periods of hunger, as can be achieved through fasting, are increasingly becoming the focus of interest.

Food with resveratrol.

Substances that mimic the biochemical processes of Lent will also help. The speech is, for example, of resveratrol. Studies have shown that this secondary plant substance from raspberries, grapes, plums, or red wine can also trigger autophagic processes in the cell. Another study even showed a connection between resveratrol and the prevention of Alzheimer's disease.

Food spermidine.

Another natural substance, spermidine, also acts on the activation of autophagy. The content is found, among other things, in various foods, such as in soy products, legumes, mushrooms, mature cheese, and wheat germ. Among other things, studies with fruit flies have shown that adding spermidine to food can counteract age-related dementia. It has also been demonstrated in an animal model with mice that the additional intake of spermidine protects heart health can. Background of the protective effects of spermidine is always that autophagic processes are intensified.

What does that mean for your body?

The cells stay healthier and, thus, the entire organism when the "garbage collection" in the cell is working correctly. It is still too early to make a final assessment of this, but there are many indications that most degenerative diseases are also the result of a tedious recycling function in human cells. As a result, both pathogens and degenerate cell components can accumulate, which over a long period causes loss of function and disorders at higher levels of the organism. Perhaps degenerative processes are, therefore, nothing other than the consequence of a disturbed renewal at the cellular level.

AUTOPHAGY
ENDOGENOUS RECYCLING

♦ ♦ ♦

Cellular building blocks for autophagy

The cells are fundamental building blocks of the organism. They are always busy developing, renewing, and multiplying. To understand how autophagy works in detail, it is essential first to understand the structure and operation of these small powerhouses.

Lysosomes - Decomposition of old and building new macromolecules

Not only in the household, but also on every level of the body must be regularly disposed of the garbage. Cells are confined to the outside by a plasma membrane. Inside is the so-called cytoplasm. This cytoplasm is watery in consistency and forms the carrier for the nucleus and various organelles such as lysosomes, mitochondria, and ribosomes. A membrane also encloses the lysosomes and contains different enzymes called acid hydrolases. These are responsible for the breakdown of fats, sugars, proteins, and nucleic acids within the cell. By dissecting and releasing these complex molecules, new macromolecules can be built up. Therefore, the lysosomes are often called the "recycling plant of the cell" designated.

Ribosomes take over the protein synthesis

The ribosome is composed of a complex combination of proteins and ribonucleic acid. In the ribosomes, protein synthesis takes place. In this case, individual amino acids are converted into long-chain polypeptides.

A ribosome represents a self-sufficient production facility for every protein to be synthesized in the body.

Mitochondria - power plants of the cells

The mitochondria are among the best-known cellular building blocks. They are often referred to as "power plants of the cells" and responsible for the energy supply of the organism.

To maintain the body's substance, the cells must maintain an active metabolism. Metabolism means the construction, delivery, and degradation of proteins, carbohydrates, fats, and nucleic acids. The mitochondria supply the necessary energy for this. However, as these are not always available indefinitely, the cells must use this resource sparingly.

In the course of evolution, they have developed a technique to disassemble all available organelles or proteins into their parts completely.

It is a self-digestion process, which causes the decomposition of products to be re-metabolized. This process of recycling is the actual autophagy.

You can simplify the process by imagining a cleansing squad that swirls throughout the body, sweeping up any damaged or unneeded proteins, viruses, bacteria, cell organelles, plaques, and other microorganisms.

When this "heap" is complete, everything is burned and transformed into vital energy. Here, a healthy balance must be maintained in this perfectly coordinated mechanism.

In a figurative sense, exaggerated cleaning would cause cell death, while disruption or incomplete cleanup can trigger serious diseases such as cancer, Alzheimer's, or Parkinson's.

THE DIFFERENT PROCESSES OF AUTOPHAGY

♦ ♦ ♦

Christian de Duve had received the Nobel Prize in 1974, among other things, for the discovery of lysosomes. At that time, the researcher had discovered with the electron microscope that various stages of decay exist in a cell, which he then described as autophagy. Today autophagy is understood as three different processes.

Pexophagozytose

This process serves to break down defective peroxisomes. These are small vesicles in the cytoplasm of the cells, which detoxify toxic metabolites derived from the processing of oxygen.

Mitophagozytose

The mitochondria in the cytoplasm are particularly susceptible to the toxic metabolites of oxygen. Thus, the lifespan of mitochondria in the cells of the liver, the main detoxification organ, is just ten to twelve days. Mitophagocytosis breaks down defective mitochondria, creating the potential for rejuvenation and cell regeneration.

Xenophagozytose

This process involves the breakdown of foreign substances that invade the organism. These include, for example, viruses and bacteria.

Autophagy under the microscope: the steps of cellular self-digestion

Researchers after Duve succeeded in detailing the individual steps of autophagy. In the cytoplasm, a double-layered membrane is first formed, the so-called phagophore. It enlarges until it encloses parts of the cytoplasm and organelles. In the process, the autophagosomes, which are entirely distributed in the cytoplasm, must be transported, which must be carried towards the cell nucleus lysosomes. For this purpose, a kind of transport rail is available.

Autophagosomes and lysosomes merge and the autolysosomes form. Here, all components are decomposed using the enzymes contained in the lysosomes.

The autophagy-lysosome pathway (ALP) is one of the major pathways for the degradation of misfolded proteins. But more interestingly, ALP is the only known way to dispose of whole organelles such as mitochondria.

After this digestion process, all usable components are released into the cytoplasm. With this process, the cells succeed in ridding themselves of all harmful elements and renewing themselves continuously.

The formation of autophagosomes never stops. A certain level of activity is always present. However, there are situations where the process is in full swing. If the organism is stressed by a lack of nutrients or harmful substances from the environment, autophagosomes are increasingly formed.

Even with a lack of food, for example, by fasting, the activity increases. In principle, the starving cells save themselves by self-digestion, as they feed on the substances formed thereby. This detoxification process protects humans from many pathogens, viruses, bacteria, and environmental toxins.

However, autophagy slows down with age. If it comes to a defect in this system, many diseases can be the result.

The genes control autophagy

Nobel laureate Ohsumi investigated autophagy with yeast cells to investigate the role of the genes involved. He selected yeast cells because they show a certain degree of agreement with the vacuoles of mammals and thus humans.

Ohsumi set about eliminating the genes that contained the blueprint for the digestive enzymes in the vacuoles. A short time later, a large number of autophagosomes filled with cellular garbage accumulated. Due to the lack of digestive enzymes, no dissolution could take place, whereby Ohsumi had proved that autophagy is genetically controlled.

He then prepared the yeast cells with chemicals that caused gene mutations and disabled specific genes. He then removed nutrients from the yeast cells and starved them out.

In intact cells, the process of autophagy

It would now run at full speed due to the lack of nutrients, and swelling of the vacuoles should be observed. Only then would the cell be able to survive despite starvation. However, since relevant genes were disabled, the process could not start, and the vacuoles remained empty.

Self-digestion and suicide of the cells are closely related

However, autophagy can also trigger programmed cell death, termed apoptosis, by the medical term. Oxidative stress is capable of initiating a cellular suicide program. Durch oxidative stress, dangerous, reactive oxygen radicals (time: oxygen species) are formed. These reactive oxygen species are produced in the mitochondria. In inflammatory diseases or as part of the aging process, however, these are increasingly provided.

Once the immune system is weakened, the cells have no way to intercept these oxygen compounds. They are released unhindered and begin their work of destruction. They damage the mitochondria both indoors and outdoors. These then release signals that lead directly to cellular suicide.

At first, the cells shrink, and the bubbles on the membrane become tight.

The DNA then breaks down, and the nucleus begins to deform.

Neighboring phagocytes react immediately and destroy the damaged mitochondria. This would otherwise emit signals that would result in programmed cell death. This is especially important in the brain. Because there it is not possible to replace once damaged cells only by cell division.

As you can see from this example, healthy self-digestion and self-killing of the cells are closely related - the latter being initiated when overall cellular stress and damage are too high.

SELF-HEALING THROUGH A FUNCTIONING AUTOPHAGY

♦ ♦ ♦

Your cell function can only be sustained if recycling works optimally. Because only when harmful material is degraded, the cell can renew itself.

This is comparable to strength training. When dumbbells are lifted, small cracks develop on the muscular level. The body is once busy after training to break down all damaged muscle fragments. At the next food intake, building blocks in the form of nutrients are again available, and the muscles are rebuilt. This is one of the reasons why, after each intensive training, there should always be a rest period so that there is time for regeneration.

However, muscle breakdown and build-up must be in balance so that cell cleansing and rebuilding work together seamlessly, and there is no restriction on cell function.

This can be applied to the entire diet. If you feed too much on a lower calorie diet or if you are subjected to rigorous fasting periods, the cells no longer receive enough energy and are restricted in their function. If this process is not interrupted by food intake, eventually the cell death will be brought about.

If you overeat, however, insulin production will be stimulated. This is one of the biggest inhibitors of autophagy. Because the surplus your cells get the message that it is not necessary to tap the body's reserves. In the cells, the degradation processes are slowed down, and self-digestion is inhibited.

Especially carbohydrates in bread, sugar, pasta, and other white flour products stimulate insulin production. Protein and healthy fats, on the other hand, are needed by the cells to replace the already degraded components with new ones. Do you take this possibility your cells, accumulates in them the " garbage " and the autophagy is slowed down - the battery is dysfunctional or may even degenerate?

Anti-aging

Fasting and exercise are sometimes the best means of anti-aging, not only because of increased secretion of growth hormone but also because of autophagy. Damaged or weak cells are broken down and replaced with new batteries. This applies to cells of all kinds and slows down aging in some ways.

immune system

Autophagy also breaks down and destroys viruses, bacteria, and other pathogens in the cells. This strengthens the autophagy of our immune system and supports this in the defense against pathogens. This is sometimes a reason why we usually feel little to no hunger during illness. The body signals that it does not want food to get into autophagy. Thus, the immune system can work better, and the body heals faster.

This is sometimes the reason why fasting is so effective against so many diseases. It naturally strengthens the immune system.

Heart Health

Autophagy also has a positive effect on our heart health and supports the health of our cardiovascular system. Some studies have been able to prove this, but the exact mechanism is not yet precise.

Brain health

Another important point the researchers have been able to confirm is the effect against dementia, Parkinson's, and other brain disorders. Although the origins may be different, an accumulation of misfolded proteins is usually the cause. These accumulate in the course of life but can be effectively degraded and recycled by autophagy. Thus, autophagy protects both preventively and treated against numerous brain diseases.

Researchers were able to demonstrate this effect, among other things, by the administration of spermidine. This ingredient comes in varying concentrations in different foods and has been proven to boost autophagy. This, in turn, had a positive effect on numerous symptoms and diseases.

Recent research also suggests that autophagy is not effective in the treatment of cancer and tumors. It fights potential malignant cells and stops cancer cell growth. However, these studies have been conducted mainly in vitro or on animals. As current but human studies are carried out, there will be some exciting results over the next few years.

AUTOPHAGY ACTIVATIONO/TRIGGER

♦ ♦ ♦

There are a few ways to support and stimulate autophagy in a natural way. Here are the proven effective methods to support the body's garbage collection. Autophagy is improved by:

Fasting/intermittent fasting

The most effective method of increasing autophagocytosis is fasting. Fasting in a variety of ways forces the body to recycle and recycle damaged cells, cell & metabolic waste, and pathogens. By the waiver of food supply, it comes forcibly.

Food/nutrition

Proper nutrition can support autophagy even after fasting. A general calorie reduction, in combination with fasting, leads to increased autophagy. Also, certain foods promote autophagy. These include:

Wheat germ

Germinated wheat contains a lot of spermidine and is sometimes the spermidine richest food there is. This substance, which was recently investigated by researchers from Graz, even stimulates autophagy in a high concentration with food. A groundbreaking discovery that inspired researchers worldwide to conduct further experiments in this regard.

Sports

Sport is another possibility that boosts autophagy. Exercise, in combination with fasting (training on an empty stomach), is the ultimate combination when it comes to maximum effect. Both together increase the impact, and the autophagy is significantly boosted.

Current research shows that fasting, such as interval fasting, can be used to stimulate autophagy in a particularly useful manner. Supplements of substances such as spermidine or resveratrol provide additional accents, while **fasting forms the basis for autophagy.** In particular, interval fasting could prove to be a practical way to integrate short periods of fasting into everyday life. Here, for example, the results of the InterFAST study will be awaited, to draw further conclusions for personal growth.

A similar effect to fasting can also be achieved by **calorie reduction in** general. For example, it is common in some cultures to eat only 80% full, instance Japan. It is not yet clear that this diet prevents disease. However, the reduced food intake can be considered favorable for both health and cell health simply because excessive food intake also causes unhealthy **stress for the body.**

It takes up too much food, accelerates the formation of free radicals and often overwhelmed the body's metabolic processes. About the cell, autophagy is also involved in these metabolic processes. With voluntary calorie reduction, the cell gains the opportunity to stimulate cell cleansing. In any case, one can imagine these processes according to the current state of knowledge.

Overdressed? Then autophagy can become too intense!

In the course of cell metabolism, waste materials are formed again and again as long as we consume food and are exposed to environmental stimuli. The healthy cell ensures that, in the course of a precise balance, that the renewal processes in the cell are in equilibrium.

Too much of autophagy is only imaginable if, for example, fasting passes into long-term **starvation.** These can be **life-threatening** at a certain point in time.

However, fasting is not designed in the strict sense of prolonged starvation, but on a limitation of food intake for a specific time. The question of too much autophagy cannot yet be answered unequivocally, even according to the current state of knowledge. It is not also clear how many hours of fasting are necessary to reactivate autophagy. For this further studies and investigations are required.

So far, there is the impression that, in particular, the common degenerative diseases of old age are due **to insufficient** autophagy.

In summary, you can support autophagy in your cells by:

1. Regular fasting and targeted calorie reduction.

2. Inclusion of certain foods that are considered conducive to autophagy.

3. Spermidine and resveratrol as a dietary supplement.

Overall, it is helpful to consider degenerative diseases that increase with natural aging, always from the viewpoint of autophagy.

WHAT IS FASTING?

◆ ◆ ◆

Man is not made for the permanent supply of food. Because our ancestors did not have a regular meal program, it was eaten what nature and hunting luck gave. Especially towards the end of winter, the supply was scarce, and most of them had no choice but to fast.

Exactly this habit has stored the evolution in the genes. Fasting is a normal process for which the body is predisposed, while it permanently burdens permanent food at regular intervals.

Numerous are the studies that demonstrate the positive effect of fasting on physical health - and on the mind. It is not for nothing that almost all world religions know regular fasting times. Fasting can help in the prevention and cure of diseases such as migraine, diabetes, high blood pressure, arthritis, rheumatism, and even cancer.

Abandonment demands a lot from the body and mind, which is why most people take a break for it. With intermittent fasting, however, there is an everyday way to health available to everyone.

What does autophagy have to do with interval fasting?

In short: the significant improvement of your health! Autophagy is more pronounced during interval fasting and reaches its peak after a fast of approximately 14 hours. Therefore, my recommendation for the 16: 8 interval fasting method, since the cell cleaning in the 16 hours really has time for cleaning AND disposal.

This way, unique (decrease) effects could be realized with ease. Here I can only let my personal training customers speak, whom I accompany and support, and who can now keep their success easy for many years.

The explanation for the improved decrease is the following: too frequent food inhibits the self-cleaning process of the cell. The cell literally "lapses" when autophagy is prevented from being purified by the constant supply of energy from the outside.

WHAT IS INTERMITTENT FASTING?

♦ ♦ ♦

Intermittent fasting, interval fasting, or abbreviated 'IF' is not a diet. You can see it better as a diet. The emphasis is not on what you eat, but on when you eat. An example: you do eat between noon and 8 pm, you do not eat the other hours. With this method, you fast 16 consecutive hours.

By fasting intermittently, you can experience various positive effects. Losing weight, more energy, increased resistance, and a boost for your brain are some of the benefits.

Build lean muscle and burn fat by not eating!

Intermittent fasting or simply intermittent (interval) fasting is a very effective means of burning fat and building muscle mass. It makes your life a lot easier because you are not busy eating all day. Fasting has numerous health benefits, but it also works wonders for your fat burning and muscle mass.

What is intermittent fasting?

The name says it all; you eat at intervals or not. Intermittent fasting is not a diet but a diet. You decide for yourself when you will and will not eat, and you choose a period of time that best fits your lifestyle. Do you work during the day, and do you have social arrangements in the evening, or do you eat together with the entire household? Then you fast during the day and only start eating in the afternoon. There are different variations to fast, but the most common method is the 16: 8 method. This means that you eat 16 hours fixed (not eat) and 8 hours. Then you have the 18: 6, 20: 4, 1 meal a day, eat-stop-eat and a few other methods.

Losing weight and building muscle

By not eating. Wait! You are not supposed to eat anything. On the contrary, you eat all your entire day in need of macronutrients but in a shorter time. In the period that your body gets no calories through your diet, fat reserves are used as useful energy for all body processes. Your metabolism (metabolism) does not decrease! In fact, fasting speeds up your metabolism. Research (see source) shows that 24-hour fasting stimulates the production of growth hormones of up to 2000%. This is extremely high, and it speeds up your metabolism. Growth hormones stimulate protein synthesis so that cells are able to grow and recover faster. Growth hormones also have a direct effect on fat cells. Fat cells release part of their content as fuel for all body processes; this is called Lipolysis. Lipolysis is nothing more than breaking down / splitting fat cells for energy. During fasting, you use your own body fat as fuel, and at the same time, you build muscle mass.

When intermittent fasting is to extend the time between meals, typically the hours between dinner and the subsequent meal the next day, the most popular and most suitable for everyday use is to forgo breakfast and have lunch again. For example, if you finish your dinner until 8:00 pm and eat again at 12:00 the next day, you will have a 16-hour fasting period followed by 8-hour food intake.

Of course, other temporal variants are conceivable. Most researchers are also experimenting with other forms of intermittent fasting, for example, eating only one meal a day (24-hour fasting), or changing one day completely without a meal to one-day eating (English every other day fasting).

THE BENEFITS OF INTERMITTENT FASTING

1. LONGER LIFE

A study among rats showed that the animals that we're obliged to do intermittent fasting lived 36% to 83% longer than those who followed an ad libitum diet (a diet where they could eat anything they wanted).

2. LOSS OF WASTE

By doing intermittent fasting, you automatically limit your calorie intake. Because of this, intermittent fasting will probably ensure that you lose weight without having to (consciously) put too much effort into it.

3. HEALTH FOR YOUR HEART

Intermittent fasting could cause LDL cholesterol, the 'bad' cholesterol, to decrease in your blood. This is better for your heart.

4. ANTI-INFLAMMATORY

A few studies show that intermittent fasting causes specific inflammatory markers in your blood to go down. Inflammation is often the cause of chronic diseases.

5. HEALTHY BRAINS

Intermittent fasting would ensure a healthier brain. Not eating regularly increases the BDNF hormone that can contribute to the development of new nerve cells.

6. INSULIN RESISTANCE

Intermittent fasting can decrease insulin resistance. Besides, it can lower your blood sugar by 3% to 6% and your insulin level by 20% to 31%.

7. DISPOSAL OF WASTE

During intermittent fasting, your body has time to start crucial cellular repair processes, such as cleaning up cell waste. This process is called autophagy.

WHY YOU SHOULD FAST REGULARLY

1. Learning to live without food

Most of us live in abundance and always have enough food in our fridge. But what happens when an emergency situation forces us to eat less, or at times, nothing to eat? How does that feel? How long can you stand this?

Anyone who has fasted once, do a meal without suffering a circulatory collapse. Man has always fasted because the food was not always and at any time in sufficient quantity. We modern humans, however, have no need for fasting and, therefore, unlearned. Your chance to make it part of your life again.

2. Discover something new (sharpen your sense of smell)

If you have ever wanted to know how the Stone Age man has found his food sources, then you should definitely fast.

Your sense of smell will sharpen, and you will again perceive odors that you have not had in your nose for a long time. The barbecue party ten houses away, suddenly seems to take place in your garden. The bouquet or a glass of red wine reveals completely new smell experiences. Yes, once you have overcome the first boring hunger, these intense smells are a real experience.

3. Purify and detoxify

During Lent, the digestive organs are allowed to rest and the liver to recover. They start to get rid of toxins and toxins and excrete them.

Of course, you do not smell like Cleopatra after a milk bath at this time, but finally, all the garbage is supposed to come out.

To support this process, you can take a hot bath, sauna, or endurance sports. Enemas, warm liver wrap, and extra sleep are also beneficial.

4. Strengthen discipline

After many years of self-experimentation, I am sure that any change in diet or any change of habits will only lead to success with iron discipline. After a week of fasting, you are, in any case, able to keep you and your appetite for junk food better in check.

From the second week of fasting, you can cook food for your children and your partner and then sit down to eat without getting tempted. Because you have a goal and that's what it's about. The smallest sin during Lent, kills everything, and subsequent stomach cramps are as safe for you like the men in the church.

5. Lose weight

The reasons for fasting can be varied, yet most people just want to lose weight. For me, it was not different at first.

Although losing weight naturally does not pose a major problem during fasting, weight loss should not be the main reason for fasting. Be aware that if you do not fundamentally think about your diet after Lent, you will have all your lost weight on your hips after a few weeks.

6. Change diet

There is no better time to change your diet than after a fasting week. Because now you have weaned yourself from solid food and cleaned your body. So, why not break with old habits and try something new?

Make an exact plan on how to proceed after Lent and get suitable recipes so that you do not fall from being without a plan, immediately back into your old pattern of behavior.

7. Getting to know one's body (getting to know the limits of one's body)

The first days of fasting are according to experience the worst. You can only think of food and not think clearly. But you will be surprised how much your body can do even if it gets no more food. For example, during my last fasting phase, I walked almost 7 km every day, and it fascinated me so much that my body did it.

This reminds me of a quote from my coach: "Most people have enough fat reserves to walk from Cologne to Moscow without taking food!"

8. Remove grease

On the third day of fasting, your body has used up its glucose stores. Of course, if you move daily, it will happen sooner. Now, he starts to attack the fat from the depots in order to gain energy from it.

By now, everyone should realize that you do not need carbohydrates to survive. The body can produce that itself. However, to provide the brain with vital energy, the body must switch from glucose metabolism to fat metabolism. This condition is called ketosis, and every person reaches this state after three days at the latest without food intake. Now the body starts to burn fat, and the pounds finally tumble. In addition to a strictly ketogenic diet, fasting is the safest way to reduce body fat.

9. Optimize drinking behavior

What brings you the greatest weight loss when it was only water in the end? Many fasting newbies realize three weeks after fasting that they have regained their old weight. The golden rule of fasting is, therefore, always: "drink regularly and drink more than usual!"

If you have drunk little water before your first week of fasting and have mostly quenched your thirst with juices, soft drinks, and coffee, then it will now be much easier for you to change your drinking habits and more or better to drink only water.

Especially during fasting, clear water helps you to eliminate hunger and keep your circulation stable. You learn to distinguish between hunger and thirst, and you will drink significantly more after the fasting week and need fewer snacks.

10. Eat more consciously / eat slower

It has been my experience that for most of us, food is becoming a necessary evil to take time for. As a result, many people eat a lot of smaller meals in between and hardly spend more time eating.

Family life often suffers from this, as children are eating almost always slower, always talking and sometimes even forget the food. No wonder they are rarely overweight.

They give the body enough time to develop a feeling of fullness.

During Lent, you will not eat solid food anymore, and the few moments you can allow yourself broth or vegetable juice are very valuable. So, you'll spend a lot of time eating or slurping and enjoying every single sip.

WEIGHT LOSS

If you are overweight, achieving weight loss through a balanced diet and regular exercise makes sense. But weight loss can also be a symptom of a disease. In principle, any illness, whether through physical or mental mechanisms, can lead to weight loss. Greater, unwanted, and inexplicable weight loss over a period of time should be clarified, especially in elderly patients. Weight also plays a major role in eating disorders.

What is the symptom?

Weight loss generally means a decrease in body weight. This may be intended as part of a diet or unintentionally as a symptom of a disease. In medicine, an unwanted weight loss of more than 10% of body weight within half a year is considered a warning signal.

An unwanted loss of weight is often not noticed at the beginning or even perceived as positive. Others push out weight loss for a fear that a malignant disease may be behind it. Eye-catching is the weight loss when the body fat reserves are exhausted, and it comes to the reduction of muscle mass: one speaks of underweight. With pronounced weight loss, there is often additional malnutrition. A very heavyweight loss in the context of serious illnesses (e.g., cancer) is called cachexia ("wasting").

In general, one differentiates a weight loss with normal or increased appetite from a weight loss with reduced appetite. In addition to unwanted weight loss, there are usually other complaints that already give clues to the cause. Examples are:

- Problematic eating behavior, such as cravings and self-induced vomiting in an eating disorder (eating, bulimia).

- Sweating, restlessness, diarrhea, or goiter at hyperthyroidism (hyperthyroidism).

- Severe thirst, frequent urination, fatigue, and poorly healing wounds in diabetes (diabetes).

- Fever and night sweat in cancer or chronic infections (e.g., tuberculosis).

- Concomitant symptoms: loss of appetite, general weakness, absence of menstruation, susceptibility to infections, gastrointestinal discomfort (nausea, vomiting, diarrhea)

What illness can be behind it?

Weight loss can have many causes, ranging from poor nutrition to physical or mental illness, alcohol abuse, or side effects.

Causes of weight loss with normal or increased appetite include:

- Metabolic disorders: hyperthyroidism (hyperthyroidism), diabetes (diabetes mellitus)

- Gastrointestinal infections and diarrhea

- Worm infections of the intestine (e.g., bovine or fish tapeworm)

- Chronic inflammatory bowel disease (e.g., Chron's disease or ulcerative colitis)

- Disturbed food use in celiac disease or gluten intolerance

- Food allergies (lactose intolerance, fructose intolerance)

- Chronic pancreatitis (pancreatitis)

Causes of weight loss with decreased appetite include:

- Chronic infections (e.g., tuberculosis, AIDS)

- Advanced heart failure (heart failure)

- Kidney failure (renal insufficiency)
- Adrenocortical insufficiency (Addison disease)
- tumor diseases
- Medication side effects
- Eating Disorders: Anorexia (anorexia), bulimia (eating-crushing addiction)
- Mental illnesses: depression, borderline syndrome
- Mental stress, stress
- self-help

A healthy lifestyle with a balanced diet, regular exercise, moderate alcohol, and abstinence from nicotine promotes good physical and mental health and helps to prevent diseases that can be associated with weight loss.

Regular check-ups (including cancer screenings) should always be performed. If a disease-related weight loss has already occurred, it is first necessary to stabilize the body weight and to compensate for the loss as far as possible — this helps doctor or nutrition expert.

When to go to the doctor?

A slight weight loss is usually harmless and is often explained by changes in dietary or lifestyle habits. An unwanted and unexplained weight loss, however, is always suspicious and should be clarified by the doctor. In particular, if in a relatively short time, a lot of weight was lost or if additional concomitant symptoms exist. An extreme weight loss due to an eating disorder (anorexia nervosa) can even lead to death if left untreated.

The normal weight is roughly defined above the BMI (body mass index) and should be between 18 and 25. If the bodyweight is 15% or more below normal weight, then medical advice should be sought.

Which doctor is responsible?

family doctor
Internist
gastroenterologist
endocrinologist
oncologist
Psychologist / Psychotherapist
nutrition expert

What does the body do in a diet with muscles?

By dieting in a diet, you specifically targeted for a calorie deficit. So, you eat fewer calories than your body consumes. By this circumstance, you decrease, because your body has to resort to its reserves.

Your body gradually reduces your existing energy reserves. This is primarily the body fat, which is degraded for this purpose and used to provide energy.

However, in such a diet, the body also relatively quickly begins to reduce "unnecessary" structures to approximate the energy requirement to the energy supply. This includes a reduction of the trained muscle mass.

Also, your body can respond to a prolonged calorie deficit with even greater austerity and hormonal changes. As a result, your muscle maintenance is severely compromised, and weight loss can be slowed or also stopped.

1) Do not eat too little

A too-large calorie deficit can quickly cause your body to take emergency measures. In this situation, robust energy consumers (your skeletal muscles!) That are not vital are reduced, and the releasable nutrients are used to generate energy.

Therefore, you should make your diet so that a calorie deficit of about 20% is not exceeded. This may take a bit longer to reach your weight loss goal, but you do not risk unnecessary muscle loss. Besides, you have the goal of sustainable fat loss with your diet, since too much deficit also greatly accelerates your hormonal conversion.

2) Supply sufficient protein

A lack of carbohydrates, your body can still compensate relatively quickly. Humans are not necessarily dependent on this nutrient. The body can extract substitutes (ketone bodies) from the body's fat reserves. Fats and proteins, on the other hand, are essential nutrients that must be fed through the diet.

The body needs protein for building up and maintaining body structures and also for the production of (sometimes vital) hormones. Proteins can also be used to generate energy. If you do not take enough protein in your diet, your body gets the protein from another place: your muscles.

For this reason, it is essential in a diet to have enough protein to create the best conditions for maximum muscle maintenance. Experience shows that athletes with a protein intake of about 2.5 g per kg of body weight can minimize the loss of muscle in a diet. Under (ambitious) bodybuilders also three and more grams per kg of body weight are recommended.

You can ensure your protein intake by choosing high-protein foods. But it may also make sense to take one or the other protein shake to supplement you.

Schedule Cheat Days/loading days

If the body gets less energy than it needs over a more extended period, it goes into a saving mode with the metabolism to adjust the energy requirement of the supply. Under these circumstances, the muscle breakdown in your diet is additionally accelerated.

To keep the metabolism up to speed, you can incorporate a cheat day (or loading day) into your diet. This means eating more calories on a given day than the body needs to suggest a surplus. This counteracts the hormonal change. Depending on diet and body fat percentage, a different frequency of application is appropriate.

Training & Fasting: So, you can combine it

Focus on muscle preservation, not build up! Your performance is limited, as new stimuli are too much for your body.

Try to train so that you have just finished showering at sunset. So, you can directly enjoy your post-workout diet - one of the most important, if not the most important meal for losing weight, gaining muscle, and defining! Here, simple carbs are not only allowed but even desired!

Shifts your rhythm as best you can: The sun sets only later - you can even lie down for an hour before the workout. That gives you power for training. Plus point: You are automatically awake longer and have more time for exercise and (healthy) feasting.

Not start with competitions!

Does without cardio, because since you sweat a great deal and your dehydrated body loses more fluid.

In any case, screw-down the intensity and the volume down. Even if you have the energy - you risk losing muscle!

Go for a full-body workout instead of your other split training. So, you can be sure that each muscle group charged twice a week, despite reduced training - this is enough for muscle maintenance. Treat yourself to more breaks than usual and do everything a bit more relaxed - even the training frequency, because more than three workouts a week should not be even for the freaks among you.

ARE ALL CALORIES THE SAME?

♦ ♦ ♦

Have you ever wondered if all calories are the same? If we go by the laws of thermodynamics, all calories are the same - at least on paper. But the way our body processes carbohydrates, proteins, and fats, and the effect that these nutrients have on our bodies are very different. We'll tell you today what nutrients work on your body and why not all calories are the same.

Fats

In addition to being a strong and tasty source of energy, fats slow down digestion and provide fat-soluble vitamins, which are important building blocks for our cells.

All dietary fats have about nine calories per gram, but as you probably already know, there are fats that are better for our body and our health than others. Polyunsaturated omega-3 fats in foods such as wild salmon or flaxseed are anti-inflammatory and protect the cells. By contrast, artificial trans fats can increase the risk of heart disease.

Proteins

Proteins saturate long-lasting as they slow down digestion. The real purpose of proteins is to care for and renew the cells in our body. Most important are proteins for children, adolescents, and pregnant women, as the cells are constantly renewed during these phases of life. But even during a diet, it is particularly important to eat enough proteins, as they saturate for a long time and protect against muscle breakdown.

All dietary proteins have about four calories per gram, but again there are differences in valence. The appetite regulates, for example, fish or eggs. These foods also support muscle recovery and are ideal as part of a diet. Lower quality proteins are found in hamburgers, for example. These are branched-chain amino acids that may be responsible for metabolic diseases and elevated insulin levels. Make sure that you consume high-quality protein, so you can get the most out of a diet.

Carbohydrates

Carbs are by far the most complex calories, as there are many different types of carbohydrates (e.g., fiber, starch, sugar), and these are processed by our body in very different ways.

Carbohydrates are used by our body like a fast source of energy and immediately provide our brain, liver, and muscles with new energy. All carbohydrates have about four calories per gram (except fiber because our bodies cannot digest them). But even with carbohydrates, there are again differences in valency.

Dietary fiber is a high-quality and important carbohydrate because it slows your digestion (you are full for longer) and prevents the absorption of other nutrients - such as sugar. High-quality carbohydrates ideally contain a lot of fiber and are only minimally processed. These include fruits, vegetables, whole grains, and legumes.

A calorie of fats is, therefore, not the same as a calorie of proteins or carbohydrates, and our body processes and utilizes these calories differently. There are also different types of sugars that are absorbed differently by our bodies. Let's look at and glucose and fructose.

Starchy foods such as rice, potatoes, and pasta are mostly made from glucose, a simple sugar that can be burned to extract energy from every cell in our body. Glucose is stored in our liver and muscles and delivers fast energy during, for example, during a workout or during sleep. Unprocessed, starchy foods such as brown rice, potato with shell, and wholegrain pasta will also contain fiber, vitamins, and minerals.

In contrast to glucose sugar - which is burned by all our energy-producing organs - fructose can only be broken down by the liver. The natural occurrence of fructose can be found in fruits, for example. With additional fiber, this source is good for your body. Unfortunately, today, we also find fructose in many processed foods.

The main difference between fructose and glucose is that too many calories of glucose can lead to a general weight gain, and less harmful adipose tissue is formed. On the other hand, too many calories from fructose can damage the liver and lead to fatty liver disease.

So, you see, not all calories are the same. As a matter of principle, you should make sure that you eat the most calories from minimal or unprocessed foods because they have a much higher quality and are better not only for weight loss but also for your health.

MACRONUTRIENTS

♦ ♦ ♦

Macronutrients are those nutrients from which the body gains energy. Carbohydrates, proteins, and fats are included. Alcohol is also assigned to the macronutrients.

All processes in the body, such as breathing, heartbeat, digestion, growth, tissue regeneration, and much more, require energy. The body has to absorb this energy via food in the form of certain nutrients - the so-called macronutrients. During their metabolism, the energy contained in them is released.

Units of energy content

How much energy a nutrient contains is given in joules (J) or calories (cal).

Joule or kilojoule (kJ) is the international unit (SI unit) for food energy. A joule equals the amount of energy required to move one kilogram with a force of one newton by one meter.

Previously, the energy content of the food in calories or kilocalories (kcal) was specified (1 kcal = 1000 cal). A kilocalorie is energy needed to heat one liter of water from 14.5 to 15.5 degrees Celsius. One kilojoule equals 0.239 kilocalories; one kilocalorie is 4.184 kilojoules.

The individual macronutrients have different energy content. One gram of fat has a calorific value of 37 kJ (9 kcal), and one gram of protein or carbohydrates contains 17 kJ (4 kcal). One gram of alcohol has an energy content of around 30 kJ (7 kcal).

However, the body cannot utilize all the energy contained in the food. About five to ten percent of food energy is excreted. In particular, proteins are not fully utilized.

How much energy does the body need?

The energy requirement of the body depends on many different factors such as age, gender, health status, climate, work severity, etc. Every human being has an individual energy requirement.

The total energy requirement of humans is made up of basal metabolic rate, output, and heat generation.

Basal metabolism

The basal metabolic rate (GU) is the amount of energy that the body needs at least to sustain all vital bodily functions such as heartbeat or respiration. It corresponds to the energy consumption of a human twelve hours after the last food intake with physical and mental rest and a constant ambient temperature of 20-28 degrees Celsius.

Power sales

The powered turnover (LU) indicates how much energy the body needs for physical activity and the regeneration of tissues.

Heat generation

The body also consumes energy during thermogenesis (thermogenesis). Heat formation is influenced by food intake and ambient temperature. If you eat, the body needs extra energy to transport and break down the nutrients it absorbs. This increased energy consumption manifests itself in the form of heat generation. The body also needs the energy to regulate body temperature. If it is cold, it produces heat, for example, by consuming energy.

They are the three main suppliers of nutrients in our diet. Our bodies receive energy through them, but they have other vital functions. These are:

1. CARBOHYDRATES

Carbohydrates are the most important source of energy for our brain and physical activity. Monosaccharides (simple sugars) are the basic building blocks of carbohydrates. One differentiates depending on chain length between:

- Monosaccharides: glucose, fructose, galactose
- Disaccharides: sucrose (table sugar), lactose (lactose)
- Oligosaccharides: raffinose
- Polysaccharides, or complex carbohydrates: amylopectin (vegetable starch), glycogen (animal starch), inulin

Carbohydrates are stored in the form of glycogen in the liver (⅓) and the musculature (⅔). The glycogen stores are available to you under physical stress and are replenished by a carbohydrate-rich meal.

The Nutrition Society recommends that adults consume at least 50% of their daily energy in the form of carbohydrates. You should prefer complex carbohydrates. They cause (unlike simple carbohydrates) no blood sugar spikes, keep you full for a long time, are rich in minerals, among other things provide fiber, have a positive effect on your gut health, and lower cholesterol levels.

THESE FOODS ARE RICH IN COMPLEX CARBOHYDRATES:

- fruit
- vegetables
- legumes
- breakfast cereal
- (Freshwater) Potatoes
- whole-grain products
- brown rice

SIMPLE CARBS CAN BE DERIVED FROM:

- Sugar
- White flour products
- Sweets
- sweetened lemonades and fruit juices

When it comes to carbohydrates, pre- and probiotics should not be missing. Regular consumption is said to have a beneficial effect on intestinal health.

2. PROTEIN

A protein consists of chain-like linked amino acids. There are a total of 20 amino acids in the body. These are classified into essential, conditionally essential, and nonessential amino acids. Essential amino acids cannot be produced by the body itself and must, therefore, be fed through the diet.

The macronutrient protein has numerous functions in the human body. Protein acts as a hormone, enzyme, and antibody in defense against infection. Furthermore, it occurs as a body structure (connective tissue, skin, hair, and muscle fibers).

Our muscles account for about 60% of the main memory for protein. However, this memory is not used directly as an energy source, but rather as a building material.

You should take about 1 g per kilogram of body protein per day. If you want to gain muscle mass, your need can increase to 1.2 to 1.8 g per kilogram of body weight. Are you strength athletes? Then you should take protein together with carbohydrates after the workout (ratio 1: 3). The intake of carbohydrates leads to the release of insulin. This has a positive effect on muscle growth through its anabolic hormonal action.

THESE FOODS ARE HIGH IN PROTEIN:

- meat
- fish and seafood
- Milk products
- eggs
- legumes
- grain products
- nuts
- soy products

A clever combination of certain foods helps to increase the biological value.

3. FAT

Fat is a flavor carrier. In our diet, lipids (fats) occur in solid (e.g., butter, coconut fat) and liquid form (vegetable oils). One distinguishes between the following fatty acids:

Polyunsaturated fatty acids also include omega-3 and omega-6 fatty acids. These are essential and, therefore, need to be absorbed through the diet. They are included in cold-water fish (salmon, herring, mackerel), thistle oil, linseed oil, and nuts. The ratio of omega-3 and omega-6 intake should be about 1: 5.

The human organism requires unsaturated fatty acids for the metabolism and elasticity of cell membranes. They also improve the flow properties of the blood and are important for the growth and regeneration of cells.

In addition to valuable fatty acids, fats also provide fat-soluble vitamins A, D, E, and K. Animal fats also contain cholesterol. From this, the body can form vitamin D through sunlight on the skin. Cholesterol is also involved in hormone production. Nevertheless, a high cholesterol diet is discouraged because it promotes the development of the cardiovascular disease.

The fat content in our diet should be around 30 to 35 %. Saturated fats should not exceed 10% of the total energy intake.

WHAT INTERVAL FAST VARIANTS ARE THERE?

♦ ♦ ♦

There are four different ways you can do intermittent fasting. The instructions are quite simple: each variant indicates how long each of the fasting phases and the food phases are. Which form suits you personally, you decide, depending on eating habits and daily routine. Beginners usually start with 16/8, advanced fast even whole days. Just test it out!

16/8 variant

In the 16/8 option, you eat your meals within 8 hours and keep your fasting phase for over 16 hours. This method is best for fasting intermittently over the long term. 16/8 also facilitates entry into interval fasting.

Example: You take your first meal at noon and your last meal at 8 pm. After 20 o'clock, you will be up until noon the next day.

36/12 variant

Anyone who gets along well with fasting and can easily manage a day without food can acquire the 36/12 option. You eat only every other day within 12 hours. For example, you eat from 8 to 20 o'clock. The next night, the following day and another night until 8 am, you are fasting, and only unsweetened drinks are allowed to be drunk. Sounds hardcore; it is synonymous for many and, therefore, a type question.

20/4 variant

Similar to 16/8, it is eaten in a 20/4 rhythm. 4 hours of food, 20 hours of fasting. This variant is also for advanced users who can live without food for a long time. For example, you take your first meal at 2 pm, and you're last at 6 pm. The next night and the morning until 14 o'clock you are fastest.

TIPS ON HOW TO START INTERMITTENT FASTING

The 16/8 variant facilitates the start

If you're looking for Interval Fast for the first time, 16/8 is the perfect way to start. Because during the day you can eat enough within 8 hours, the fasting phase goes on during the night, where you sleep anyway and do not have to think about it, if you should maybe have a snack against the small hunger. If you find the 16/8 variant easy, you can gradually switch to one of the other variants and even take full days of fasting.

Persist: The first days are the hardest

As a warning, the early days are the hardest. Because it may be that the transition is difficult for you initially if you are used to eating a meal late at night or need a hearty breakfast very early. Hold on, because after a few days, the feeling of hunger disappears during the fasting phase, and you notice the positive effect the new rhythm has on your performance. Until then, always remember, appetite is often a matter of the mind. The more you think about food, the higher the desire for it. In the first few days, it's best to steer clear of sports or other activities and drink water or tea as soon as you get hungry.

Sport promotes fasting success

Sport is good anyway and supports your success in intermittent fasting. Because the movement metabolizes your last meal faster, your glycogen stores are emptied, and you get into the fasting phase and thus into the ketosis more quickly. Sports in the morning before the first meal speed up the process also.

Do not eat sugar!

You want the full benefit of interval fast? Because let sugar in every way. Because sugar provides glucose, your plan in intermittent fasting, however, is to promote ketosis. And the more sugar your body gets, the less it pulls its energy out of the fats. Healthy foods are the prerequisite for interval fasting to increase your strength and brainpower. This means that sugar and fast food are taboo and carbohydrates should be eaten for the optimal effect also possible only in small quantities. You can eat your fill of fish, meat, eggs, and vegetables.

INTERVAL FASTING:
INSTRUCTIONS FOR THE 16/8 VARIANT

♦ ♦ ♦

The better you prepare for interval fasting, the easier it will be for you. Here are some tips:

Set mealtime

Important for the 16/8 variant is the rhythm of 16 hours fasting/eating 8 hours. Think before you: Are you the type who prefers extensive breakfast and instead of dinner without a meal? Or do you not need to eat immediately after getting up in the morning and wait until noon with your first meal? Accordingly, you choose your food rhythm, e.g.

- 9 am an early meal, 5 pm last meal or
- 12 o'clock first meal, 8 o'clock final meal.

You set the start time according to your eating habits, 8 hours later you should then eat the last meal of the day. Since the digestion goes down after 10 pm, you should finish your mealtime at 9 pm at the latest. The late-variant is even advisable since the morning of the fast-benefit is more excellent. Then fat burning and hormone production work exceptionally well. So, if you're one of the breakfasts, you should gradually postpone your first mealtime to lunchtime for even more. Make sure you think about it - it's worth it!

Allowed drinks during fasting

Drinking is permitted during fasting! It should be the right thing, though. Water is always and at any time, as well as unsweetened herbal tea and ginger tea. A cup helps wonderfully when a feeling of hunger arises. Unsweetened coffee and green tea are also ok. However, not in the evening, as they can make you sleep with caffeine.

Create interval fasting plan

The better you prepare for your daily routine, the easier it is for you to get started and also to hold on to the interval. Therefore, make a plan with food and meals that you always have at hand until you have developed a specific routine. Here's an example of when you've decided on a midday start for 16/8 fasting:

- **Morning:** After getting up, it's best to cover the hours until your first meal with tea or coffee. Even a bulletproof coffee or butter coffee is allowed because it contains no carbohydrates and supports by the contained MCT oil the ketosis.

- **First meal:** Your first meal will be available at noon. No matter when you eat your first meal, it's best to be low carb. At noon, a combination of proteins and vitamins, such as salmon and spinach or avocado.

- **Afternoon snack:** To be efficient in the afternoon and to prevent food cravings, you can eat a handful of nuts or a bite of nuts and fruits.

- **Last meal:** At 8 pm, you end your mealtime with a protein-rich snack, combined with vegetables. Here you can make e.g., an egg omelet. This is quickly prepared and provides you with proteins.

NUTRITION PLANS FOR INTERMITTENT FASTING

Intermittent fasting works best with a nutritional plan that you prepare in the early days. Such plans you can put together on the Internet for free. Recipes help you to maintain your diet during intermittent fasting and to resist the temptations of high-carbohydrate snacks. Here are a few suggestions for the first days:

Recipes for breakfast:

In the fasting phase, your metabolism has just slowly switched to ketosis - because you do not want to bring it back with carbohydrates back to the glucose recovery. That's why we prefer a Bulletproof Coffee or a protein shake, for example, for breakfast

- 1/2 avocado
- 1 handful of spinach
- 200 ml almond milk

- 1 tbsp coconut oil
- high-quality protein powder
- possibly water for consistency

If you prefer something to bite, an omelet with spinach and tomato is a tasty alternative:

- 2 eggs
- 1 spring onion
- 1 handful of fresh spinach
- 1 tomato
- 25g of feta
- salt and pepper

Fried egg with bacon and stir-fried mushrooms is almost a breakfast classic:

- 3 eggs
- 3-4 strips of bacon
- 200g mushrooms
- Chives or parsley

Recipes for lunch or dinner:

A mix of proteins and vitamins is still your best friend, so there is also lunch and dinner a combination of fish or meat and vegetables, e.g.

Chicken breast with spinach and feta

- 120g chicken breast
- 250g of spinach
- 50g feta
- 1/2 onion
- 1 clove of garlic
- 2 tablespoons rapeseed oil
- salt and pepper

Dice onions, press garlic and sauté briefly in the oil. Add spinach. Season the chicken and fry in oil. Then season the spinach and crumble the feta over it.

Salmon with vegetables

- 150g salmon
- 1 zucchini
- 6 cherry tomatoes
- 1 spring onion
- 1/2 clove of garlic
- 1 dash of lemon juice
- some thyme
- 1 tsp olive oil
- salt and pepper

The preparation is super easy: put baking paper on a plate, spread the vegetables on it, but the salmon on top, drizzle with herbs, spices, lemon, and oil. Then form a packet from the baking paper and cook it at 180 degrees for 20 to 25 minutes in the oven.

Zucchini noodles with tomato sauce and shrimp

- 1 zucchini
- 200g passed tomatoes
- 1 teaspoon tomato paste
- 1 clove of garlic
- 1 tsp olive oil
- 150g shrimp
- salt and pepper

Cut the zucchini into small strips with the vegetable peeler and leave to simmer for 1 to 2 minutes in boiling salted water. Prepare the tomato sauce, let the shrimp grow in it, and pour over the zucchini noodles.

20: 4 interval fasting

20: 4 interval fasting, also known as **Warrior diet,** is another method for the increasingly popular interval fasting. It is a kind of aggravated version of the 16: 8

method (also known as fasting for 16 hours). With this, you fast for sixteen hours and eat in a time window of 8 hours. At the 20: 4 interval fasting, you will consequently be able to fast for 20 hours and eat in a 4-hour time slot.

This diet was invented by Ori Hofmekler, who had the "warriors" (Warrior) of the early days in mind: These spent many hours everyday hunting for food and had to provide excellent physical services. Eaten only once in the evening by the fire with the trunk - but then large portions. Intermittent fasting is based on this understanding.

This is how 20: 4 interval fasting works

The Warrior diet reduces the daily food intake window to 4 hours. In these four hours (this should be the evening hours), then in detail is fed as much as the refrigerator gives. In the other 20 hours, food intake does not have to be eliminated. Just as the warrior paused while wandering around the country, smaller amounts of dairy products (e.g., a cup of yogurt), fresh fruits and vegetables, as well as protein-rich snacks such as hard-boiled eggs and nuts, maybe eaten during the day. Also, plenty of low-calorie drinks such as water and tea should be drunk.

Most people fast during the day and place the four-hour window for eating in the early evening hours. But here, too, everyone has to find out for himself which time window fits best. You can consume two meals or a more substantial dinner during this time. Others eat a lunchtime meal around 12 or 1 p.m. and a more significant supper at 5 o'clock before the time window closes. You have to decide for yourself, which times work better for Interval fasting for you. It's usually easier to avoid food during the day as you are distracted with work, sports, and other activities.

Being active in sports does not hurt

Analogous to the warriors who used to roam nature for many hours to hunt animals, you should be as productive as possible during the Warrior diet during the day. Of course, this is not so easy if you have to spend the day at the desk. Try to exercise, for example, during lunch or in the late afternoon before the four-hour window for eating. After the meal, you should not do any sports anymore. The body comes to rest in the evening and then focuses entirely on food and digestion.

Even with the 20: 4 interval fasting, your food should always contain wholefood and protein-rich meals, i.e., you should focus on meat, fish, eggs, vegetables, and fruits and use carbohydrates only sparingly. Here are the recipes on our site delicious.

Fasting for 20 hours is not always easy

The most obvious challenge of the Warrior diet from our point of view is that you are only allowed to eat 4 hours a day. That may not be a problem on certain days. But on other days this is undoubtedly difficult. Our experience here is that, especially in ordinary life and social activities, the 20 hours fast is a big hurdle and requires the right amount of self-discipline. An invitation to brunch or dinner together can be a challenge. Who wants to sit next to it and eat nothing?

Again, it is essential still that you to have to find out for you if 20: 4 interval fast is what suits you best. Try the Interval fast with the gentler 16: 8 method, and if you realize you can handle Lent well, try out the beefier Warrior diet. That's how we did it, and it worked well. However, we must also say quite frankly that the restriction was too high for us and we, therefore, prefer the more flexible 16-hour fasting.

Some people do not like the warrior diet that much

Eating only 4 hours a day is a diet, not all people should follow. This is rather critical for the following groups of people:

- children
- People with eating disorders
- Pregnant or breastfeeding women
- People with underweight
- athlete
- People with certain diseases (diabetes 1, heart problems or similar)

Since fasting for 20 hours has a not inconsiderable influence on the human hormone balance, this method is also considered to be critical for women.

This approach can lead to eating disorders

Let us be honest with ourselves. Of course, we want to eat enough food in four hours a day. Many foodstuffs, in contrast to healthy eating habits, warn nutritionists to hurt your eating habits. Eating only large portions can cause an eating disorder. It is, therefore, important to continually question yourself critically and to observe your eating behavior well.

Other side effects were also observed

As with other changes, the Warrior diet can also cause side effects, including:

- Laziness / low energy
- Low blood sugar
- Fatigue
- Slight dizziness
- Anxiety/Depression
- Extreme hunger
- Hormonal imbalances
- Fast irritability

In our view, it's just important to listen to yourself and your body. If it does not go away, then you should consult a doctor or limit the periods in which you fast.

What's the best way to start with the Warrior diet?

There are two ways to get started in the 20: 4 Interval fast. We tried the first variant ourselves. Here we first started with the 16: 8 method, and only when we had a good feeling, the Lent was extended to 20 hours.

A second variant is the recommendation of Hofmekler himself. This recommends the start in the 20: 4 interval fasting through several weeks with different eating priorities to facilitate. The intention is to get the body used to use fat as an energy reserve faster.

The first week (also called detox week)

- This week, you should not eat much in the 20-hour window, but you should not fast. Here you should eat vegetable juices, clear broths, and dairy products such as goat cheese.

- In the 4 hours you eat, for example, a healthy salad with oil vinegar dressing. After that, you can have large or several smaller meals with vegetable proteins (for example, beans) with smaller portions of cheese and cooked vegetables.

- It is allowed to drink tea, water and smaller quantities of milk at all times.

The second week (also called High Fat Week)

- This week, you should not eat much in the 20-hour window, but you should not fast. Here you take vegetable juices, clear broths, and dairy products such as goat cheese to you.

- In the 4 hours, you can also eat a healthy salad with oil vinegar dressing. After that, you can eat large or several smaller meals with pure animal protein, cooked vegetables, and a handful of nuts.

- This week, nothing is eaten with wheat or starchy foods (corn, beans, potatoes, etc.).

The third week (cycle week)

This week, you switch between times of high carbohydrate or high protein levels.

- One or two days with high carbohydrate content

- This is followed by a day or two of high protein and low carbohydrate levels

- Again, a day or two with high carbohydrate content

- Yet, one or two days with high protein and low carbohydrate content

When you're done with the three weeks, you can start all over again. In this way, the body learns faster, as he can gain energy from fat reserves. A critical point here is that there are no portion sizes or calorie plans on the Warrior Diet.

When you switch to the regular 20-hour fasting rhythm, that's up to you. The important thing is, you feel comfortable in the approach, and your hunger attacks are not too strong.

What can I eat - what can I drink?

20: 4 Interval Fasting allows you to drink low-calorie drinks like water, (black) coffee and tea during the day, and even snack snacks like a handful of nuts, a piece of fruit, or a protein shake. Nevertheless, 20 hours is a very long time for fasting. Supporters of this diet report that by not eating, they feel more energized and fitter during the day as the body uses the non-fasting Interval fasting time to detoxify and burn fat.

Whether all this is true, of course, is questionable. Who can say today whether the warriors of the early days did not take any food supplies on the hunt or in between killed a small animal and consumed it in a more extended break? Also, a physically active hunter whose mind was focused on finding, hunting and killing animals wasted much less thought on the needs of the body than the modern desk warrior, using only Excel spreadsheets and PowerPoint presentations wrestles and always has mental idleness.

INTERMITTENT FASTING: LEANGAINS METHOD

❖❖❖

Lenten phase and food window at Leangains
In general, the fasting phase should be started in the evening, as nothing is eaten at night anyway, and continued during the next morning. Ideally, this phase ends in the afternoon or a little later.

This is true for most people who get up at 6 to 7 o'clock in the morning. The afternoon and evening are then spent with a full stomach. Depending on preference, the food window can also be started later, especially for people who tend to get up later and stay active longer in the evening.

The recommendation to go through the early part of the day in fasting is mainly socially motivated. Most people find it easier to stop eating after waking up and go to bed in the evening. From the afternoon until the evening, the window of time for food intake extends. The feasibility has proven to be advantageous with a food window in the latter part of the day.

Carbohydrates/protein/ fat, and how many calories?

Carbohydrates, Protein, Fat, and Kcal Content: These variables are mainly determined by the user's goals. Fat loss, muscle building, or body recomposition.

Basically, the amount of protein is constant - no matter what day. Such as:

- On training days, there are more carbohydrates and less fat.
- On regeneration days the other way round: fewer carbohydrates, more fat.

Four different Leangains protocols, depending on your requirement which are listed below.

The choice of the right protocol depends mainly on the intended time of training. Depending on whether 1-3 meals are provided after training.

1) Training (12-13h) in the fasting state

Strictly speaking, the training is not carried out in the fasting state. This would be counterproductive. The intake of protein, with its stimulating effects on protein synthesis and metabolism, is an indispensable measure to obtain optimal results.

Therefore, it is important to take 10g BCAA or a similar amino acid composition (e.g., 30g whey protein) on an empty stomach before training.

After training, the 8-hour meal window begins.

Example:

- 11.30-12.00 or 5-15 minutes before training: 10 g BCAA
- 12-13: Training
- 1 pm: Post-Workout Meal (Biggest Meal of the Day).
- 4 pm: Second meal
- 9 pm: last meal before the beginning of the fasting phase

Calories and carbohydrates are continually reduced over the three meals. This means most carbohydrates and calories are delivered immediately after exercise.

2) Early morning training in fasting

- 6 am: 5-15 minutes before training: 10 g BCAA.
- 6-7 clock: Training.
- 8 o'clock: 10 g BCAA.
- 10 o'clock: 10 g BCAA
- 12–1 pm: big post-workout meal (biggest meal of the day). Beginning of the 8-hour meal window.

- 8–9 pm: Last meal before the fasting period. Attention: On days off, you do not have to take any BCAAs.

3) A pre-workout meal (3 pm - 4 pm)

This is Martin's recommendation for the younger ones who can still go to school or work out at 3 pm-4 pm through flexible working hours.

Example:

- 12–13 pm Speak lunchtime: pre-workout meal about 20-25% of daily calories
- 15-16: Training, a few hours after the pre-workout meal
- 4 pm-5 pm: post-workout meal (biggest meal of the day).
- 20-21 clock: Last meal before the fasting phase

4) Two meals before training (between 5 pm and 8 pm)

This method will be ideal for most people who are tied to normal working hours.

- 12-13: First meal // 20-25% of the daily kcal requirement
- 16-17: Pre-workout meal // about the same as the first meal
- around 6 pm: training

- 8-10pm: post-workout meal (biggest meal)

Important points:

- During the fasting phase, no calories are added. Coffee, calorie-free sweeteners, or sugar-free chewing gum (up to 20g) are allowed (even if little calories are included). A small shot of milk (1 tablespoon) in the coffee has no negative effects.

- Lent is perfect for getting things done and productive.

- The frequency of meals during the meal window is not relevant. Most, however, find three meals most enjoyable.

- Most of the daily calories are consumed in the post-workout phase. Depending on which of the four methods mentioned above, this means 95-99% (method 1), 80% (method 3) and 60% (method 4)

- The food window should be kept reasonably constant as the hormonal circuits adjust to the food frequency. We tend to get hungry when we are used to eating. If the food window extends from about 1 pm to 9 pm then try to keep it there every day.

- On regeneration days, the first meal should be the biggest - unlike the training days when the first meal after a workout is the biggest. Good value for this meal on regeneration days is 30-45% of the daily kcal requirement. This meal should be very high in protein. (up to 100g protein - e.g., 500g chicken breast fillet)

- If you want to save the biggest meal of regeneration days for the evening (because, for example, a celebration is due), that's fine, too. Thus, larger meals together are no problem.

- Recommended dietary supplements: multivitamin, fish oil, vitamin D, and calcium (especially if milk products are not consumed regularly).

- 10g BCAA can be replaced with 30g whey protein.

- Which method of the four described above is the best depends on the circumstances of life? Anyone who works in normal working life with working hours from 9 to 17 o'clock - with the only possible time training after working - usually goes with method four best. Running Method 1 with this schedule tends to be a bad idea.

16: 8 INTERVAL FASTING: THE 8-HOUR DIET

This is how interval fasting works in 16: 8 time

- Eight hours a day are there to eat, 16 hours fast.
- Drink at least eight glasses (about two liters) of water a day.
- Give up fast food. Eat what is really filling for a long time.
- Always combine two power foods with each meal.
- Coffee is taboo after 14 o'clock.
- Just a glass of wine a day (if at all)
- Do sport for at least eight minutes every day, of course, more.

For whom the Interval fast is suitable

Think about how the eight-hour eating period fits best into your daily routine. For early risers, it is advisable to move the first meal of the day to 9 o'clock, but then dinner will take place at 5 o'clock. If you work longer, you should start with the meal only in the morning (at 11 o'clock) and can plan the dinner for 19 o'clock.

No matter which option you choose, **there are no rigid eating rules and no-calorie restriction in the selected eight hours.** "You can eat what tastes best and what you feel like doing right now." That's what makes the 16: 8 weight-loss method so great: This form of interval fanning is suitable for everyone and can be integrated into everyday life.

Move before breakfast!

For our bodies to burn as much fat as possible, what we eat at what time of the day is decisive.

It's over after eight hours

If you put dinner forward, your glycogen stores will be empty, and the body will burn more fat during the night. "It's crucial that you really do without nibbles in front of the TV because otherwise the slender effect is gone," emphasizes the expert. " **Focus on three main meals, if** you whip out the snacks altogether, you'll gain more muscle mass."

An example daily routine for interval fasting

- 7 o'clock: get up. Short workout
- 8 o'clock: Drink two glasses of water.
- 10 am: Time for a hot drink to boost your metabolism (coffee or tea).
- 11 am: Breakfast, e.g., muesli with fruits
- 13:30: Lunch, e.g., a wholegrain sandwich with salad and ham
- 2 pm: last chance to drink coffee (caffeine stays in the body for 8 hours)
- 17 clock: Now is the best time for sports! Studies show that with activity before 20 o'clock, 22 percent more muscle mass is built up.
- 6:30 pm: dinner. Now put on good fats and protein. If you like to drink a glass of wine, then now - later consumed alcohol disturbs sleep.
- 19 clock: Last chance for a sweet dessert (like two ribs of chocolate!) Before the 16-hour fasting period
- 11 pm: Go to bed.

AUTOPHAGY RECYCLING AND SURVIVAL

♦ ♦ ♦

Humans have learned to build recycling plants only in recent decades. Biological cells have mastered the principle of waste disposal and recycling for billions of years. Today, cell biologists are familiar with two degradation pathways through which defective or excess cell components return to the material cycle. In so-called proteasomes, a cell breaks down smaller debris such as peptides and proteins. The process of autophagy or autophagocytosis is more responsible for the larger structures, such as protein complexes or even whole organelles such as mitochondria and ribosomes. In doing so, a cell not only disposes of waste resulting from defective fabrication, UV radiation, or heat. Autophagy is a so-called constitutive process, meaning that it is continuously running at a low level. But in times of hunger, the machinery suddenly works at full speed.

Relevance to Alzheimer's and cancer?

On the purely morphological level, cell biologists already understand the recycling processes quite well. Organelles or protein complexes that are to be degraded enter the cell interior in a so-called autophagosome. This is a bubble, which is covered by two membranes. The autophagosome melts during the process with a so-called lysosome. It contains enzymes that can break down cell components; This cell compartment breaks up the debris into the molecular parts. But how does the cell know which structures it should break down? How exactly do autophagosomes arise? Also, which molecules mediate and control the entire process?

All questions that are also of medical relevance, because autophagy plays a vital role in many diseases. The protein aggregates that are deposited in the brain of an Alzheimer's patient (so-called plaques) arise because, among other things, the process of autophagy no longer works properly. Also, cancer cells also play a role in recycling, even in the twofold sense: cells in the outer regions of a tumor must block the process. Otherwise, they digest themselves and die (autophagy can ultimately also be lethal and, in addition to apoptosis, be programmed Cell death type II). Cancer cells in the center of a tumor, on the other hand, are cut off from the nutrient supply and have to digest themselves to a certain extent in order to keep alive.

Every hunger has its consequences

They ask which proteins and signal molecules play a unique role when the cell increases its autophagosomal activity. With the method of mass spectrometry, they scan the entire arsenal of proteins that are formed in the cell, the so-called proteome. They compare cells that "self-digest" at a reasonable level with cells whose autophagosomal activity is elevated. To do this, they must expose part of their cells to a real bottleneck; For example, they reduce their amino acid intake. "If certain proteins are produced in particularly high quantities after such starvation, they may play an important role in the process of autophagy," says Dengjel. Another approach is to find proteins, who suddenly suffer from hunger stress phosphate groups. Such proteins are likely to play an essential role in the signaling process surrounding autophagy, as phosphate groups transfer from signal molecule to signaling molecule in cellular signal cascades and activate the next step in a single pathway.

For a long time, biologists thought that autophagy was a nonspecific process. They assumed that an autophagosome eats everything that gets in its way. Dengjel and his team have shown with their work that this cannot be. After a 36-hour shortage of amino acids, for example, the researchers from Freiburg observed that not all proteins and cell components are broken down at the same speed. In the proteome of the cell, parts of ribosomes and molecules necessary for protein biosynthesis disappear first; The battery does not need them because amino acids are missing anyway for the building of proteins.

Molecular backgrounds and work in the system

Is there a lack of amino acids? Lipids? Carbohydrates? Or does the cell need to dispose of defective components after damage caused by chemicals? The composition of the proteome of cell changes depending on these "stimuli." "We can pretty well rule out that autophagy is nonspecific." It is probably even the opposite. Other researchers' work shows that there is a specific process of autophagy for each type of organelle: mitophagy for mitochondria, reticulophagia for endoplasmic reticulum, or bibliography for ribosomes.

AUTOPHAGY HELPS FIGHT ALZHEIMER'S

♦ ♦ ♦

Why is that so important?

We know that autophagy plays a role in many diseases. We can get infections if autophagy is not working correctly, but we can also use autophagy to repair the damage. The next step is to find out how we can influence and counteract diseases. This is a whole new field of research. That was not possible until Ohsumi gave us this knowledge and tools.

In which diseases does autophagy play a role?

In any case, in cancer and neurodegenerative diseases such as Alzheimer's and Parkinson's. But also, in inflammation and infectious diseases, in type 2 diabetes - in many diseases that we get instead when we age.

How can we, for example, better fight Alzheimer's with Ohsumi's findings?

In many of these diseases, proteins accumulate in the brain. This is toxic, and you want to get rid of it. We know that autophagy tries that. If we can strengthen that, we may be able to reduce the symptoms of Alzheimer's.

The Nobel Jury often finds it challenging to confine itself to three candidates, as Alfred Nobel's will envisages. This time you even managed to make out only one thing.

It's unusual for a person to dominate a field of research for so long and do so much of the necessary work. When Ohsumi started his research, very few people became interested in autophagy. That's why he worked almost alone for decades. But it is unusual for a single person to leave such a mark. It was not hard to commit to him.

KETOGENIC DIET AND INTERVAL FASTING

♦ ♦ ♦

Ketogenic diet and interval fasting - what are the advantages of this combination? If you think now: for God's sake - even more complicated? Basically, it is not complicated to combine these two nutritional methods. They even go very well together, and the effect is great because they take advantage of both forms and decrease even faster and lose primarily body fat and hardly any muscles.

Studies prove that the combination of keto and interval fasting is the nutritional form where the body fat percentage is lowered the most.

The advantages of both diets at a glance:

Benefits of a ketogenic diet:

- Fast weight loss and body fat reduction
- Increased mental and physical performance and endurance (through more even energy supply than carbohydrate metabolism)
- Keeps blood sugar levels steady and prevents cravings ago
- Better concentration through "ketosis" (ability to use ketone bodies for energy production)
- Balance blood pressure and lower high blood pressure
- Reversing type 2 diabetes
- Cure migraines
- Control of epilepsy and reduction of medication
- better skin appearance, reduce inflammation and pimples
- Decrease stomach pain & nausea
- Reduce tachycardia

Advantages of interval fattening:

Reduced :

- Overweight
- Difficulty concentrating
- Headache in the morning
- Dyspnoea (shortness of breath) under stress or even at rest

- Insomnia (falling asleep and staying asleep)
- daytime sleepiness
- performance limitations
- aging process
- Cardiovascular diseases
- Cancer and Alzheimer's

Improved :

- Recovery of genes and body cells
- Blood sugar levels
- Insulin resistance
- Stops diabetes type 2
- Condition
- Regeneration
- More power during training
- Growth of new nerve cells
- Brain function and our memory

Autophagy replaces those components of a cell that have become obsolete.

The disused cell parts are renewed at the subcellular level.

How exactly did Yoshinori explore Ohsumi? The Japanese scientist found an increased number of lysosomes (constituents of cells that destroy the material) in the liver cells of rats after the infusion of glucagon. Destroyed subcellular parts and unneeded proteins are labeled and then transferred to lysosomes to finish the work. He began his work with yeast cells and found the same processes in mammalian cells as well. His studies are among the most cited works in the field of cell biology. His fundamental findings were the starting signal for the study of intracellular processes.

The special effect of autophagy on a low carbohydrate diet

The trigger of autophagy is food deprivation, so fasting. The hormone insulin is released during ingestion and increases with the absorption of carbohydrates. At the same time, the opponent to insulin, the glucagon remains low. As insulin increases, glucagon decreases. However, if insulin remains low due to adequate nutrition, the glucagon may increase.

This increase in glucagon occurs not only during fasting but also during carbohydrate restriction. A high-fat and low-carbohydrate diet lowers insulin, increases glucagon, and causes fat burning. This diet favors autophagy.

Of course, the most effective is fasting. Whether you miss out on a meal, do not eat for 12 hours, or stop eating for a day, all of this acts as a trigger for autophagy. Human genes have adapted to the fact that food was not available at all times. In times of lack of food, the metabolism was able to resort to degradation products. That fasting is salutary and has a cleansing effect, also known as the big world religions.

Fasting has a double effect. First, autophagy eliminates all old and used proteins and cell parts. At the same time, fasting stimulates growth hormones that instruct the body to produce new building blocks for the body. In the state of fasting, it not only comes to cleansing but also to complete renewal.

If you are fed up with your old kitchen cabinets and buy new ones, you must first dispose of the old ones. Only then have new space. The body works similarly. First, make room, then install new material. The order is important. Longer phrases without food create room for renewal and are the prerequisite for good metabolism. In this way, fasting can stop the aging process and possibly even reverse it. Cell debris is removed and replaced with new material. Undrawn garbage that accumulates in the cells is responsible for many aspects of our civilization, diseases, and premature aging.

WHAT AFFECTS AUTOPHAGY?

Food switches off this self-cleaning process. High glucose levels (blood sugar levels) increase insulin and lower glucagon. Even small amounts of amino acids (leucine) can stop autophagy. Diets that result in calorie restriction also interfere with the process of autophagy.

Of course, it's about balance. Too much autophagy is just as bad as too little. This brings us back to the cycle of life. Celebrate and fast! No long-lasting diets! Life needs balance. Cell renewal needs nutritious food and fasting.

The mechanism behind fasting and the keto

Fasting, like the ketogenic diet, also produces ketone bodies. That is, both principles use fat as fuel to generate energy. When we fast, we are always in ketosis. The difference is that we have no choice when fasting the body, but to take one's own stored fat as a fuel source, while we in the keto diet our body fats **also** offer from food as an energy source. So, we are in ketosis without fasting.

In other words, when we feed ourselves ketogenic all, we are in a kind of "pseudo-fasting," because here too our body is made to create ketone bodies from fats because glucose is not available because we consciously contain this source in our body,

The combination is so effective **because fat burning, ketone production, and physical well-being intensify** as we merge the ketogenic diet with intermittent fasting.

Each tool has many advantages

Fasting promotes autophagy, which means the sorting out, the dismantling of diseased, and broken body cells. In addition, during autophagy, the pathogens and invaders of the body system are detected and switched off.

Then, fasting has the added benefit of promoting growth hormone, which helps build healthy cells and mitochondria and regenerate the body. What powerful features, right?

The healthy keto, as I recommend it, has many other benefits. By integrating a low carb diet with a significant increase in the proportion of healthy fats and leafy greens in the diet, we are adapting the body by learning to favor fats as fuel. This creates a steady "stream" of energy for our everyday lives and for accomplishing our tasks. Our mind clears, and we have more focus. The brain is supplied with clean energy; we feel in a good, mental condition, and much more.

Fasting can function in this process as a "catalyst" or put it bluntly: it takes on the task of "shock" when a two-stroke engine is started cold?

What's the biggest hit with fasting plus keto?

Suppose you start with a ketogenic diet and incorporate larger amounts of fats into your eating plan than ever before. You adapt, your body learns to use these fats as fuel (by denying it the supply of carbohydrates) to make ketones.

Then, on some days of the week, you start intermittent fasting, which means you opt for an 8h mealtime window and a 16h non-food window on those days. You do that because you've already taught your body to accept fat as fuel and because it makes you feel great.

The moment you integrate fasting, your body is already so effectively focused on fat as a source that it has no choice but to go over without shrugging into the fat-burning of body fat deposits to continue to produce ketones.

You have a big advantage: your body does not choose the muscle tissue as an energy source during fasting!

ALL THE BENEFITS OF KETOGENIC NUTRITION AT A GLANCE

Here are some advantage of the keto diet:

1. 24h fat burning

In ketosis, the body is burned on fat 24 hours a day. Ketosis is the best fat metabolism workout you can do!

2. Increasing libido

Especially men react to the increased fat consumption (high-quality fat sources) with a rising testosterone level and an increasing desire. The quality of life increases.

3. Increasing stamina

Here, athletes benefit; because in endurance sports (aerobic intensity range), the body prefers to burn fat. And if fat burning in the ketosis runs smoothly, it also increases exercise endurance and endurance during exercise . Therefore, the ketogenic diet and sports are excellent.

4. Sharp focus

Some beneficial hormones (e.g., serotonin, GABA, growth hormone) are increasingly produced in ketosis. Also, ketones release more energy gram by gram than energy from glucose.

The consequence: The brain has more energy available. You feel increasing attention and focus. You benefit from work or at university.

5. Easy weight loss

Who wants to lose weight, must burn fat. In ketosis, fat is burned 24 hours a day.

With this fact and the other benefits of ketosis, weight loss is more comfortable, unnoticed, faster, and longer-lasting than most other weight loss strategies.

6. Good mood

Especially by the increased formation of GABA and serotonin report most "Ketarier" of a better feeling. And again, the quality of life increases!

7. Better sleep

The body regenerates in sleep and recovers from the hardships of the last day. Also, the brain processes information.

Since ketosis brings more energy to the brain, grams of grams, and many "garbage collection programs" in the body in ketosis get going; most Ketarians report a declining need for sleep and better sleep quality.

Healthy sleep is essential to the body!

8. Stable blood sugar

The blood sugar is constant throughout the day, as no carbohydrates are fed through the diet, fewer carbs are formed in the liver, but also hardly any are burned.

As a result, blood sugar is stable throughout the day; insulin is needed only in minimal quantities. Anyone who suffers from unstable blood sugar levels (including people with diabetes) also benefits in this regard.

9. Less hunger and appetite

Due to the stable blood sugar, the high saturation by the food, and the changed hormonal situation, most Ketarier report of less hunger, thirst, and cravings. So, your thoughts do not circle the food all day.

10. High saturation due to ketosis

Due to the high content of fat and fiber in the right recipes is always achieved a high level of saturation. A high level of satisfaction, of course. Why?

Fiber swells in the stomach and intestine bind water and lead to good saturation via activation of so-called mechanoreceptors in the stomach (registration of a full stomach).

This works in a similar way to fat: Not only does it make fat content, and it tastes perfect; in the gastrointestinal tract, there are also receptors for fat, which lead to a release of hormones (e.g., peptide YY) to saturation.

A diet or diet that makes you feel full and satisfied after every meal? Not bad, right?

11. Increased energy consumption in ketosis

Energy consumption also increases slightly in ketosis, which supports those who want to lose weight. The Bulletproof Coffee fits in perfectly here.

12. Cellular garbage disposal

Due to the low insulin levels and the moderate protein consumption, the body and every single cell in the body increasingly starts the so-called cellular garbage collection (autophagy, mitophagy, and pinocytosis).

In these difficult-sounding terms, the body breaks down old and broken. This usually happens only during fasting, but also in ketosis. Old cells, but also old components of otherwise healthy cells are degraded and replaced by new ones. A spring cleaning throughout the body!

13. Increased HDL cholesterol

The "good cholesterol" that prevents cardiovascular disease, HDL cholesterol is increased in a well-performed ketogenic diet (healthy fat sources) . The ketogenic diet is thus more and more suitable for improving cardiovascular health.

14. Lowering blood pressure

Because ketones also have all sorts of chemical effects in the bloodstream and reduce oxidative stress in the body , they have also been proven to lower blood pressure. All the hypertensive patients would benefit, as well.

15. Anticatabolic

Due to the only moderate protein consumption and negligible carbohydrate consumption in ketosis, many athletes fear losing muscle. This will not be the case, however, if the calorie deficit is not too big (or there is no calorie deficit).

Because ketones also have an anticatabolic effect in the body. From evolution, this also makes sense because, in times of food shortage, you lose valuable muscle. The agency would not do that. Instead, he sacrifices the bacon reserves during ketosis.

16. Allergy problems

Unexplained mechanisms also calm the immune system in ketosis. An allergy is an overreaction of the immune system to a non-hazardous foreign particle. These reactions are much rarer in ketosis, and allergic symptoms can be actively addressed.

17. Nutrient-rich

A healthy ketogenic diet with lots of vegetables, fish, and other unprocessed foods is very nutritious and healthy. A deficit of certain minerals or vitamins you will not have to worry about.

18. Anti-epileptic

About 100 years ago, the ketogenic diet was first used medically. Patients were epileptic children. In a pure diet, so severe ketosis, an extreme decrease in epileptic seizures were observed.

It is quite conceivable that ketosis is also very successful in children with ADHD since the underlying biochemical mechanisms are very similar.

19. Scientifically supported

More and more studies prove the efficacy of ketogenic nutrition in all kinds of applications. The reviews will convince even more and hopefully more people of the significant effect in the next few years.

STRENGTHEN MITOCHONDRIA: CELL TRAINING FOR MORE ENERGY

♦ ♦ ♦

What are mitochondria?

Mitochondria - the power plants of the cells - are small cell organelles that are responsible, among other things, for the production of ATP (adenosine triphosphate). ATP is the energy source that all our cells need to function properly. For each cell, you have not just one mitochondrion, but thousands, each of which is individually dependent on the cell's energy needs.

Like the body, which is in constant decline and build-up (Katabol and Anabol), mitochondria are also in an ongoing process of replication, consumption, growth, or degradation. The greater the energy requirement of a cell, the more mitochondria are formed and vice versa.

Why should we strengthen our mitochondria?

The ATP is formed by the mitochondria from the known macronutrients "carbohydrates" and "fats," whereby the burning of glucose (carbohydrates) for mitochondria is considered to be energetically "easier."

However, "glucose oxidation," i.e., the burning of glucose, produces more free radicals than fat burning.

Therefore, the aging process of the mitochondria is accelerated by this type of energy. Obsolete mitochondria are gradually losing the ability to burn fatty acids effectively and are increasingly relying on glucose for energy.

This can lead to a vicious circle since the self-destruct process is driven by glucose-free radicals resulting in faster and faster. The resulting consequences include high dependence on sugar and carbohydrates as well as increasing fat deposits.

As one grows older, the body's ability to produce energy effectively is compromised - whether this is the cause or the characteristic of the aging process has not yet been conclusively clarified. Some neurodegenerative diseases, diabetes mellitus, cancer, cardiovascular disease, and obesity are diseases in which mitochondrial damage may be significantly involved.

It is assumed that environmental influences and diseases can even mitigate or completely destroy the function of mitochondria and thereby worsen the energy supply of the cells and organs. This phenomenon is called "mitochondriopathy."

How do we multiply mitochondria?

If the energy requirement increases or the energy supply in the cells decreases, a special protein becomes active, which protects the cell and increases energy production (in addition, the multiplication of the mitochondria can be "arranged").

In other words, a cell reacts flexibly to external environmental influences, such as food shortages, because it must always be guaranteed a certain minimum ATP production to ensure the survival of the organism.

The name of this particular protein is AMPk. It serves as a sensor for the current energy status of the cell. Together with Sirt1, AMPk activates the so-called PGC1-alpha. A protein responsible for the growth of mitochondria and activates genes responsible for lipid metabolism.

The basic requirement for healthy mitochondria and ATP formation. For the production of ATP - i.e., energy - enzymes, calcium, magnesium *, and phosphorus are important.

The enzymes contain iron and can only be formed if there is a sufficient amount of it in the body. If in doubt, you can check your iron values with the doctor.

Calcium and phosphorus are usually absorbed sufficiently by the diet. However, if the vitamin D value is too low, it can lead to a disruption of the absorption of calcium and phosphorus in the intestine. This can lead to a possible undersupply.

Magnesium is another important component of energy metabolism. For this reason, I always add enough magnesium. A magnesium compound that can be well absorbed by the body and purchased at very low cost is magnesium citrate, or even better, a combination of magnesium citrate and bisglycinate.

With which biohacks can you strengthen your mitochondria?

How can we use this knowledge with the help of biohacking and put it to practical use?

1st cold training

To freeze the body - be it the cold shower or ice baths. The idea of putting the right stimuli through cold training and training the body on a cellular level inspires me.

The many hormonal and health benefits are very convincing. It has also been found that the cold training

PGC-1 can be induced, which stimulates the mitochondrial biogenesis and respiration in the muscle cells in several ways.

In addition, chemical or cold thermogenesis plays a greater role in regular exposure to cold. This is the fat oxidation in brown adipose tissue. This adipose tissue is particularly pronounced in babies and is increasingly falling back in adulthood.

The cloud: In contrast to white adipose tissue (abdomen, buttocks, etc.), this adipose tissue has a large number of mitochondria, which directly oxidize the fat and thus generate heat.

Despite regression, it has been found in many studies that this brown adipose tissue can be reactivated and thus plays a major role in the body's heat production.

2. Altitude training for mitochondria

High altitude training is a form of exercise that is widely known among sports teams and competitive athletes and is characterized by an "oxygen-poor training environment." The low oxygen saturation ensures that, among other things, changes in the cardiovascular system, respiratory system, and the blood system take place.

For example, in mountainous regions, native Tibetans have ten times as much nitric oxide (NO) in the blood as people living just above sea level. This high nitrogen monoxide enrichment leads to a doubling of the blood flow compared to German conditions and to an optimized supply of oxygen.

But let's get back to the mitochondria. In fact, we find interesting adaptation mechanisms of these small energy donors also in altitude training: after just minutes and a few hours, they show changes that are far ahead of those of blood formation.

They adapt to the environmental influences, so as to keep the body in a physiologically beneficial area. Among other things, it has been found that altitude training increases the mitochondrial ability of fatty acid oxidation, fat burning.

If an optimal load range is maintained in altitude training - also hypoxia training - the adaptation process of the mitochondria proceeds in such a way that an increase in performance results.

3. Endurance training strengthens the cell power plants

Endurance training promotes the formation of new mitochondria in the muscle fibers. When we recall the mechanisms of mitochondrial regeneration, the following conclusion is only logical. As the energy demand of the cell increases, more mitochondria must be formed to increase the "oxidative capacity" and provide enough energy.

But beware: Taking antioxidants after physical exercise can reduce mitochondrial biogenesis.

It is also interesting that physical training promotes not only mitochondrial biogenesis in the muscle cells but also that many new mitochondria are formed in the brain.

The reason may be the high energy expenditure of the brain for motor control.

4. Calorie restriction

As you already know, the body builds new mitochondria if it cannot produce enough energy, or if its energy needs increase. By calorie restriction, we can wonderfully artificially produce this lack of energy.

In a large observational study, the inhabitants of Okinawa were investigated because they wanted to find out why the people there live so long. The special thing about this region is that four to five times as many centenarians live there as in other industrialized countries.

During this observational study, it was found that residents consumed about 20% fewer calories than the rest of Japan.

Longevity genes such as Sirt1, which could be activated by this calorie restriction and is involved in mitochondrial biogenesis, among others, were found more frequently in these people.

However, this type of diet also has unpleasant side effects. In a high-calorie diet, the bone mass decreases, the muscle strength decreases, and there is a significant reduction in sex hormones and thyroid hormones.

Dietary supplements

And because biohackers often act on the principle of "little effort and great utility," I've compiled a list of potent agents to increase mitochondrial density and efficiency for you:

Alpha Lipoic Acid - Part of the nootropic "Solid mind Focus" Alpha Lipoic Acid promotes mitochondrial function, reduces oxidative damage, and increases metabolic rate.

PQQ - PQQ has not been known for a long time and was only discovered in 2003 "as the first vitamin in 55 years". Among other things, it increases the growth and energy production of the mitochondria.

Coenzyme Q10 (Ubiquinol) - CoQ10 is essential in energy metabolism and is produced by the body itself. With increasing age, however, the CoQ10 concentration continues to decrease. When supplementing with food: Ubiquinol (a form of CoQ10) has a much higher bioavailability than the conventional Ubiquinone, which can be found in cheap CoQ10 preparations.

Resveratrol - Resveratrol has long been the figurehead of the wine industry and the reason for claiming that a glass of wine is healthy during the day. In fact, resveratrol has shown similar life-prolonging effects and mitochondrial responses to calorie-restricted diets, even with high-calorie diets. (For this reason, red wine is far from healthy, because the negative properties of alcohol overshadow the benefits of resveratrol).

CIRCADIAN RHYTHM

◆ ◆ ◆

Circadian rhythm or circadian rhythm (in Latin circa "around," "approximately" and this "day" as well as Greek ρυθμική rhythmiké or ρυθμός rhythmós "rhythm") is called in chronobiology the endogenous (internal) rhythms, the one-period length of about 24 hours. This term was introduced in 1959 by Franz Halberg. He is often Germanized today, the circadian rhythm is written and popularly known as the "inner clock."

Basic features

Although the biological background and mechanisms for circadian rhythms are different between different organisms, the circadian rhythms have specific characteristics common to many different species. The exact period length can vary between different species but is usually 22 to 25 hours. The inner rhythm does not need any signals from the outside world to follow its rhythm, which is not always exactly 24 hours long. However, the process can adapt to a precise 24-hour cycle by being able to correct itself with the help of external stimuli, the so-called timers. This process is called synchronization.

The external stimuli that can serve as timers are different for different species, but the most important and perhaps best known is the light. Other timers are, for example, temperature, and social stimuli (z. B. alarm).

Another feature of internal clocks that are not fully understood so far is that they are not affected by the organism's pH or body temperature. Changes in ambient temperature may be a sign of morning or evening effects for some species. Although almost all known chemical reactions occur faster at higher temperatures, the periodicity in the organism is independent of temperature and pH.

Why you should look for a healthy circadian rhythm

The mechanisms behind your inner clocks

Have you ever wondered why you get tired in the evening? Or why your stomach growls every day at the same, predictable time? The answer to these and many other questions lie in our circadian rhythm. Every living thing, from the tiny bacterium to insects, to complex mammals like us humans, has internal clocks that help to tailor its biological processes to the demands of different times of the day.

The internal clock of the human being is transmitted through the hypothalamus of the brain, also called the suprachiasmatic nucleus (SCN)is called synchronized and kept going. This area of the brain receives information about our environment, such as the intensity of ambient light, and processes it to accommodate our innate inner rhythms. Thus, we stay biologically on course and do certain activities at the right time. For example, the brain releases the hormone melatonin in response to diminishing brightness so we can fall asleep more easily. Melatonin also stimulates cell repair that works best when we rest. When we look for a healthy circadian rhythm, we are prepared for the challenges of everyday life, and important biomolecular processes can take place at the right time.

Why is a healthy circadian rhythm important?

While our bodies are designed to synchronize our inner rhythms with the environment, modern life can be challenging. Many people work at unusual times; others have a job that requires frequent travel, which is why jet lag occurs. Many of us spend most of our time indoors, away from stimuli such as daylight and temperature, giving feedback to our circadian rhythm. Also, our environment is usually so bright that those parts of our brain that control our inner clocks get confused.

An irregular circadian rhythm can make sleep impossible even though you are exhausted because the body is uncertain when it is time to sleep and be awake. If this is the case over a longer period, it can seriously affect your health. People whose circadian rhythm is not well regulated are at greater risk for a variety of diseases. Certain types of cancer occur more frequently, which may be due to the lower melatonin level. In addition, they suffer from higher levels of triglyceride, which is why atherosclerosis and cardiovascular diseases are more common. A dysregulated circadian rhythm also has a pronounced effect on metabolism. Therefore, these people are more likely to develop diabetes, insulin resistance, and many other common metabolic problems. Sleep is so important to human health, which is why sleep deprivation has been declared a carcinogen by many major health organizations.

Sleep hygiene: How to keep your inner clocks intact

Of course, the inner clocks must be regulated. This is often easier said than done. Fortunately, good sleep hygiene can be the solution for many sufferers. Sleep hygiene refers to behaviors that promote good night sleep. These measures are not very specific in detail, but together they can result in a healthier circadian rhythm. Consider changing the following factors if you want to make 2019 the best year ever for your inner clocks.

Keep to a regular schedule, go to sleep at the same time every day, and get up at the same time, even on weekends. Deviations of more than 20 minutes can cause a dysregulated circadian rhythm. Avoid napping, if possible, as you will be more awake at night. Turn off screens in your bedroom, including TVs, computers, and other devices such as smartphones. Use your bed only for sleeping and for sexual activities. All other things, such as lying awake and worrying, should be relocated to another location. This will help your brain to connect your bed to sleep rather than other activities.

Limit your caffeine intake to the morning hours. Drinking caffeinated beverages afternoon makes you more alert, even hours later, when you go to sleep.

Move enough at the right time - for most people, the optimal time is before 14 o' clock. Develop a soothing routine at bedtime. Take a warm bath, drink a cup of herbal tea, or otherwise relax each night. This will help you strengthen your circadian rhythm, become calmer, and be ready for sleep.

Short-term oxygen reduction could reset the circadian rhythm.

Reducing oxygen is generally considered bad for health. However, a new study suggests that this could reset the circadian rhythm of a human for a short time.

Many people have suffered from jet lag at some point in their lives. The cause is simple: a circadian rhythm disorder. To cure jet lag is much more complicated and often requires a days-long, slow adaptation to the new sleep-wake cycle. However, a recent study in the field of chronobiology suggests that reducing oxygen for a short time could reset the circadian rhythm and thereby quickly cure both jet-lag and other circadian sleep disorders.

When mice have jet lag

Even though mice do not travel across multiple time zones, they still suffer from jet lag. Just like humans, they too can experience differences in their environment, such as summer and wintertime, as well as a changing temporal sequence. Also, the metabolism of rodents (including how much oxygen is consumed) varies over a 24-hour day.

Those symptoms that jet-lagged mice will experience will be familiar to people who have had the disorder: fatigue decreased cognitive function, and sleep problems. However, when rodents are administered lower levels of oxygen for a short time immediately before a significant disruption of their circadian rhythms, they appear to adapt almost immediately without the usual side effects of a jet lag.

HIF1α and the oxygen demand of a cell

The researchers quickly determined that HIF1α is the protein responsible for this response to the low oxygen environment. HIF1α is a protein that tells cells how to use oxygen and how much of it to use. It also appears to be involved in several other cell processes, many of which depend on oxygen. Mice in which the gene for this protein was deactivated did not respond to changes in oxygen level with a recessed circadian rhythm, as was the case in normal mice.

Could low oxygen levels reset the human circadian rhythm?

Human life is generally more complex than that of mice. We have a variety of problems with our circadian rhythm, from jet-lag to shiftwork. A disturbed circadian rhythm has been implicated in diseases such as type 2 diabetes or heart disease. Also, jet lag can cause discomfort in people, as they have to adapt for days to the change. This is comparable to changing working hours and even with the time change.

Since humans also have this protein, their health could have a significant impact. For example, they could pull a mask over their face and inhale air with low oxygen levels for a few minutes, but only so long that no health problems arise.

Do not try this at home

Although promising, you mustn't use it as a home remedy. Too little oxygen can be dangerous unless it is carefully planned and used. Until scientists find a way to make this method available to the public without hesitation, you should follow any measures that have proven useful, such as melatonin, light therapy, and other safe methods to help you reset your circadian rhythm.

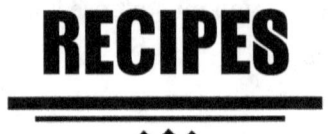

CAULIFLOWER PIZZA

Pizza is one of the most popular dishes in the world, so it is even better if you do not have to do without it during a diet. This ketogenic diet recipe is for a simple salami pizza.

Of course, you can also choose a different topping, just make sure that your ingredients also contain as few carbohydrates as possible. This recipe is designed for a whole tin of pizza and produces six pieces.

PER PIECE: 264 KCAL (19G FAT, 8G CARBOHYDRATE, 15G EGG WHITE)

1 whole cauliflower
100g Parmesan
1 egg
15g almond flour (you can use this for example)
50g canned tomatoes chopped
100g grated Emmentaler (optional mozzarella or another cheese can be used)
50g salami
2 tbsp olive oil
Italian herbs
salt

pepper
PREPARATION:

Cut the cauliflower, cut the florets, place in a blender and chop until a fine powder has formed. Place the cauliflower powder in a microwaveable container and fry for 4 min at the highest level.

Then put on a kitchen towel and let cool well. Now comes the most important step: the steamed cauliflower must be thoroughly squeezed out with the kitchen towel until no excess liquid comes out.

In a bowl mix the Parmesan, 30g of the Emmentaler and the almond flour. Then add the cauliflower and the egg as much as possible, mix the mixture, season with a spoonful or with your hands and with salt, pepper and the Italian herbs.

THE DOUGH IS NOW DISTRIBUTED ON A PAPER SHAPED PAPER, PRESSED AND PRESSED FOR 15-20 MINUTES AT 220 ° INTO THE OVEN UNTIL THE DOUGH IS EASILY GOLD-BROWN.

For the topping the chopped canned tomatoes (optional is also ready-made pizza sauce, but make sure that no sugar was added) on the dough and season with Italian herbs, salt and pepper.

Also distribute the remaining Emmentaler and salami on

the dough. Now the pizza comes back in the oven for about 10 minutes until the cheese has melted and it is as brown and crispy as you want it to be. Finally, add the olive oil over it.

EGG SALAD

Eggs are true all-rounders and hardly dispensable during a ketogenic diet. Egg salad is also a quick and easy recipe that is perfect for lunch at work or as an uncomplicated dinner.

In addition, it is very versatile and can be easily adapted to the various tastes. You can also prepare a larger portion, then you have something for the next day. You can simply eat the egg salad on its own or use it as a dip for vegetables such as chicory or cucumber.

418 KCAL (23G EGG WHITE, 6G CARBOHYDRATE, 33G FAT)
3 boiled eggs
1 avocado (about 130 g)
50 ml of water
1-2 teaspoons curry powder
salt
pepper
Lemon juice of a lemon

PREPARATION:

Puree the avocado with the lemon juice, water and spices until a creamy sauce has formed. If it's too creamy for you, you can dilute it with a little more water. Cut the boiled eggs into small cubes and mix with the avocado sauce.

Optionally, you can also add some mustard or 1-2 tablespoons of vinegar, if you like it a bit sharper. Instead of avocado you can also use mayonnaise. When buying mayonnaise, you just have to pay attention to the carbohydrates that are not too many.

FRITTATA

The frittata, an Italian omelette, is another way to use eggs. It can be prepared quickly and easily.

602 KCAL (39G EGG WHITE, 6G CARBOHYDRATE, 45G FAT)

3 egg
30g cream
30g bacon cubes
50g feta cheese (or another cheese like Emmentaler or goat's cheese)
30g fresh spinach
100g cocktail tomatoes
salt
pepper

PREPARATION:

Dice the sheep's cheese and cut the spinach into thin strips. Whisk the eggs with the cream, salt and pepper. Mix the spinach and eggs and place in a heat-resistant, greased dish. Garnish with the feta cheese, the cocktail tomatoes and the bacon and bake for about 30-40 minutes at 180° in the oven until it has solidified.

COOKING WITH ZUCCHINI

PRO PORTION 640 KCAL (38G EGG WHITE, 8G CARBOHYDRATE, 49G FAT) (TOTAL RECIPE MAKES 3 PORTIONS)

1 tbsp coconut oil
500g minced meat mixed
600g zucchini
90g cream
150g canned tomatoes
45g Emmentaler
salt
pepper
Garlic at will
Italian herbs

PREPARATION:

Fry the minced meat in a pan with the coconut oil. Then add the canned tomatoes, the cream and the spices.

Slice the zucchini. Now, in a heat-resistant container, alternately layer a layer of zucchini and a layer of minced meat. Finally, sprinkle the cheese over it and bake the casserole for 30-40 minutes at 180 ° ready.

MINCED MEAT CASSEROLE WITH ZUCCHINI

640 KCAL PER SERVING (38G PROTEIN, 8G CARBOHYDRATES, 49G FAT) (TOTAL RECIPE GIVES 3 SERVINGS)

1 tbsp coconut oil
500g minced meat mixed
600g zucchini
90g cream
150g canned tomatoes
45g Emmentaler
salt
pepper
Garlic at will
Italian herbs

PREPARATION:

Fry the minced meat in a pan with the coconut oil . Then add the canned tomatoes, the cream and the spices.

Slice the zucchini. Now, in a heat-resistant container, alternately layer a layer of zucchini and a layer of minced meat. Finally, sprinkle the cheese over it and bake the casserole for 30-40 minutes at 180 ° ready.

GOAT CHEESE IN BACON ON SALAD

Salad is best suited for ketogenic recipes, as it contains, for example, lamb's lettuce at 100g below 1g carbohydrates, but it looks like a huge portion. However, so that you do not remain unsatisfied after the meal, it can be refined with delicious toppings, such as here with goat's cheese wrapped in bacon.

695 KCAL (29G PROTEIN, 7G CARBOHYDRATES, 62G FAT)

1 teaspoon of coconut oil
80g corn salad
40g rocket
80g goat cheese
50g bacon strips
1 tbsp olive oil
1 tsp mustard
2 tablespoons white balsamic vinegar
salt
pepper

PREPARATION:

Wash and clean salad and rocket and arrange on a large plate. For the dressing, mix mustard, vinegar, oil , salt and pepper . If necessary, dilute with a little water and then pour over the salad.

Slice the goat's cheese and wrap it with the bacon. Fry the goat cheese in a pan with the coconut oil until crispy and arrange on the salad. Finally, grind freshly ground pepper over it and serve.

BROCCOLI CREAM SOUP

This soup is perfect for preparing a larger portion. Simply double or triple the quantities. For example, you can freeze the rest, so you always have a ketogenic meal ready.

351 KCAL (8G PROTEIN, 7G CARBOHYDRATES, 31G FAT)

1 tbsp coconut oil

200g broccoli

50g cream

300 ml vegetable broth

PREPARATION:

Cut the broccoli into small pieces and sauté with the oil in a pot. Add the vegetable broth and cook the broccoli until soft. Add the cream and puree the soup. Season with salt and pepper .

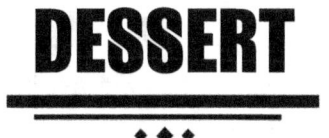

COCONUT PRALINES

Especially at the beginning of a ketogenic diet, it can be difficult to reach the necessary amount of fat to avoid starvation. These delicious chocolates help.

The nutritional information varies depending on the type of chocolate you are using. In this recipe, this form was used, a praline is equivalent to about a tablespoon.

111 KCAL PER PRALINE / PER TABLESPOON: (1G PROTEIN, 0.4G CARBOHYDRATES, 12G FAT)

200g coconut oil

2 tablespoons of almond paste (for example this one here)

2 tbsp coconut (for example this one here)

100g chopped almonds

Stevia (eg Borchers Stevia liquid table sweetener)

ground vanilla (eg Azafran vanilla powder)

PREPARATION:

The oil with coconut and - almond give in a pot and slowly melt. The vanilla stir and as necessary with stevia sweet.

Pour the liquid into silicone molds and distribute the chopped almonds evenly over all molds, then chill for at least 1 hour. Then push the chocolates out of the mold and store in a lockable container in the fridge.

AVOCADO PUDDING

The idea of preparing avocado sweetly may irritate one or the other at first. However, the creamy consistency and the taste of the avocado go perfectly with the chocolate.

597 KCAL (8G PROTEIN, 12G CARBOHYDRATES, 60G FAT)

1 avocado (about 130g)

200g coconut milk (eg One Nature organic coconut milk)

12g cocoa powder (baking cocoa without added sugar)

Stevia (eg Borchers Stevia liquid table sweetener)

PREPARATION:

Puree the avocado with the remaining ingredients.

CHEESECAKE

Despite a diet you should be able to enjoy life. The less you feel you have to change everything, the sooner you will stay on the ball. So if you have guests during the ketogenic diet or are invited for coffee and cake, just back this cake.

Hardly anyone will realize that he is without carbohydrates and you can enjoy eating cakes because of your diet.

230 KCAL PER PIECE (WHOLE CAKE = 10 PIECES) (12G PROTEIN, 3G CARBOHYDRATES, 19G FAT)

300g cream cheese

525g quark

6 eggs

Stevia (eg Borchers Stevia liquid table sweetener)

ground vanilla or vanilla flavor (e.g. Azafran vanilla powder)

PREPARATION:

Mix all ingredients, add stevia as needed and place the dough in a greased springform pan . Bake for 60 minutes at 150 ° top and bottom heat. Then allow to cool well.

KETOGENIC BREAD

For bread lovers, however, there are some clever recipes to bake a delicious, completely carbohydrate-free bread. Here is one of them.

Ingredients:

1/2 cup almond flour

2 tablespoons of coconut flour

1/4 cup of golden flaxseed

1 1/2 teaspoons baking soda

5 eggs

1/4 cup of coconut oil

1 tbsp honey

1 tablespoon of apple cider vinegar

PREPARATION:

Mix almond flour, coconut flour, linseed, salt and baking powder with a food processor.

Add eggs, oil, honey and vinegar and knead well.

Place the dough in a greased coated bread pan (or lined with baking paper).

Bake at 180 ° for about 40 minutes.

Allow to cool and serve.

Ketogenic brownies

Ingredients

20 g butter
20 ml Sunflower oil or coconut oil
40 g Xylitol (sugar replacement)
20 g Chocolate (xukcolade), noble bittersweet
2 Egg (he), separated
20 g Back cocoa
1 / 4 TL bicarbonate of soda
1 pinch salt
1 pinch cinnamon
1 pinch Vanilla, fresh
70 g Almond (s) with shell, ground

PREPARATION:

Working time: approx. 15 min. / Cooking / baking time: approx. 25 min. / Level of difficulty: simple /

Preheat the oven to 180 ° C top / bottom heat.

Separate the eggs. Beat the egg white with a pinch of salt and set aside. Then melt the butter, oil and xukcolade together. I do that in the microwave. Then mix all ingredients, except for the egg whites, with the butter-chocolate mix / mix. The crowd gets pretty tight. Carefully fold in the egg whites.

In a best with baking paper or aluminum foil designed small form fill. Can be baked as a cake or brownies. Depending on the mold height and oven, bake for 20 - 27 minutes. Do a chopstick test.

Note: This is the best ketogenic cake I have ever eaten. It is not mushy and does not taste like sweetener etc. It tastes just like a delicious almond nut chocolate cake. Serve either neat or with melted xukcolade or almond shards.

Salmon rolled over by bacon, with spicy vegetable pan and feta cheese

Ingredients

125 g Salmon fillet (s)
50 g Bacon
100 g broccoli
100 g mushrooms
70 g zucchini
70 g Feta cheese or goat's cheese or your choice
10 g Parmesan, grated
1 pinch salt
1 pinch pepper
1 pinch chilli flakes
1 pinch paprika
1 Onion (n)
5 ml Peanut oil or olive oil

PREPARATION:

Working time: approx. 15 min. / Cooking / baking time: approx. 12 min. / Level of difficulty: normal

Wash salmon and pat dry. Wrap completely with bacon. Clean, wash and cut broccoli, mushrooms, onions and zucchini.

Place a coated pan over medium heat and add oil. Add

salmon with bacon and the prepared vegetables to the pan, season the vegetables with salt, pepper, chilli flakes and paprika. Put the lid on. Just before the end of the roasting time (about 10 minutes) add feta to the vegetables. Garnish and add the parmesan to the vegetables.

Tip: For larger amounts of fish and vegetables should be best done in different pans.

Lemon Muffins

Ingredients

110 g Mascarpone, or butter
6 m. –Large (S) Egg
5 tbsp Sweetener (Huxol), liquid
400 g Almond (s), blanched, ground
1 m. –Large Lemons)
1 / 2 kl. Bottle / n Aroma (lemon)
1 kl. Bottle / n Butter-vanilla flavor
1 pck. baking powder

PREPARATION:

Working time: approx. 15 min. / Cooking / baking time: approx. 25 min. / Level of difficulty: simple

Separate eggs and beat egg whites until stiff. Mix the remainder, then carefully stir in the egg whites. Pour dough into 16 muffin cases and mix between 20-30 min. bake at 170 ° C. Make a stick sample.

100 g have only about 2.8 - 3 g of carbohydrates.

Variation:

Use 2 tablespoons of cocoa powder (no sugar, not the instant beverage) and 1 tube of rum flavor instead of the lemon and lemon flavor. Makes delicious chocolate muffins. Here you can also take the normal ground almonds, which are ground with the shell, since the dough can be dark.

Juicy strawberry cake without flour and sugar

Ingredients

80 g Butter (willow butter) or ghee
4 big ones Egg (he) (organic)
1 pinch sea-salt
15 g Xylitol (sugar substitute) for the soil
150 g Almond (s), ground
1 teaspoon, heaped Vanilla powder (bourbon)
7 g Cream of tartar
80 g cream
500 g Strawberries, ripe
1 pck. Gelatin, red or cake
2 g Xylitol (sugar substitute) for the font

PREPARATION:

Working time: approx. 30 min. / Cooking / baking time: approx. 30 min. Rest period: approx. 1 hr. / Level of difficulty: normal / calorie p. P.: about 289 kcal

Preheat the oven to 180 ° C (top / bottom heat). Melt butter or ghee gently.

Separate the eggs and beat the egg whites with the pinch of salt until stiff (overhead test). Beat the egg yolks with 15 g of xylitol until frothy. Whisk with cream and butter. Mix the almonds in advance with vanilla and tartar and also add. Then carefully lift the egg whites under the dough so that it stays fluffy.

Lay out the springform baking tray with baking paper and grease the edge well. Carefully pour in the dough, spread evenly and bake for about 30 minutes. Allow the cake bottom to cool. You can bake the soil well the day before and keep it in cling film in the refrigerator to process it the next day.

Cut the cake bottom into 8 pieces. Wrap the springform edge with cling film and place it around the bottom as a "cake ring".

Clean the strawberries, remove the green and halve the fruits if necessary. Covering the bottom of the cake without covering the cut edges, it can be easily cut again later.

Prepare gelatine or cake based on 2 g xylitol instructions. Distribute the mass evenly over the strawberries. After hamming the mass, carefully remove the springform edge.

Keep the cake cold until it is consumed. To release the aroma, remove from the refrigerator 15 minutes before. Serve with whipped cream with fresh bourbon vanilla.

Parsley root soup with green cauliflower and Stremellachs topping

Ingredients

100 g Parsley root (s), cleaned
200 g Cauliflower, if possible, greener
1 small Shallot (s), about 30 g
1 teaspoon Coconut oil for frying
700 ml water
1 Bouillon cube (organic) for 0.5 l broth, pay attention to little sugar
100 g sour cream (10% fat), dodge coconut milk in Paleo diet
Something Parsley, freshly chopped, about 5 g
100 g Smoked salmon

PREPARATION:

Working time: approx. 25 min. / Cooking / baking time: approx. 15 min. / Level of difficulty: normal / calorie p. P .: about 153 kcal

Cut the peeled parsley root and the cleaned cauliflower into small pieces. Peel the shallot and finely dice.

Heat the coconut oil in a medium saucepan and sauté the vegetables in it. Add 700 ml of water, add the bouillon cube and simmer with the lid closed for about 15 minutes until the vegetables are cooked.

Remove the pan from the heat and finely puree the vegetables in the broth. Mix in 100 g of sour cream or coconut milk with the blender.

Arrange the soup on two deep plates. Decorate with the chopped parsley.

Skin the Stremelachs and cut into small pieces to serve as a topping to the soup.

Tip: If you want to save KH, let the sour cream or coconut milk away or used instead of the brewing cube a herbal salt for seasoning!

www.ingramcontent.com/pod-product-compliance
Lightning Source LLC
Chambersburg PA
CBHW060832220526
45466CB00003B/1073